Psycho-Social Approaches to the Covid-19 Pandemic

"This book will stand as an intriguing record of 'lived experience' during the pandemic seen through a psychosocial lens. It distils this by a focus on trauma and resilience. In particular, it shows how our relationships to identity, to time, rhythm and continuity of being are disrupted, and consequently, the ways we suffer, omnipotently seek to defend ourselves, or open up to loss, strive for reinvention and forge a new orientation for new conditions."

—Chris Nicholson, *Head of Department, Psychosocial and Psychoanalytic Studies, University of Essex*

Athanasia Chalari
Eirini Efsevia Koutantou

Psycho-Social Approaches to the Covid-19 Pandemic

Change, Crisis and Trauma

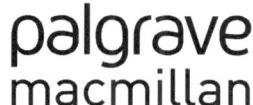

Athanasia Chalari
Hellenic Observatory
London School of Economics
London, UK

Eirini Efsevia Koutantou
University of Essex
Colchester, UK

ISBN 978-3-031-07830-9   ISBN 978-3-031-07831-6   (eBook)
https://doi.org/10.1007/978-3-031-07831-6

Cover Illustration: Lightboxx / Alamy Stock Photo

This Palgrave Macmillan imprint is published by the registered company Springer Nature Switzerland AG.
The registered company address is: Gewerbestrasse 11, 6330 Cham, Switzerland

The original version of the book has been revised. Incorrect spelling of the author's name Anathasia Chalari has been corrected to Athanasia Chalari. A correction to this book can be found at https://doi.org/10.1007/978-3-031-07831-6_7.

This work is dedicated to each of our families, each of our sons and husbands who have motivated, inspired, supported, encouraged us and rather unintentionally gave us purpose during the Covid-19 Pandemic.

Foreword—A strange situation

Pascal wrote: 'I have often said that the sole cause of man's unhappiness is that he does not know how to sit quietly in his room' (Pensées 136, p. 67). He seems to be speaking about a capacity to sit with ourselves, perhaps even *within* ourselves, and to contemplate our situation. Staying at home during coronavirus may, over time, have helped some of us to become more aware of interiority. Without the stimulus of the external world the busy mind might search inwardly. Desire to travel, explore and map both the geological and social world, itself travels inwards instead mapping the terrain of the internal world. Hence there was, during the lockdowns, an increase in contemplative activities—writing, painting, reading, taking up new skills, and exercise. The need for solitary exercise meant that many people took up running—which seems like an external activity but is more often in fact, a solitary confrontation with our essential nature—we run with our minds as much as our bodies. In all these ways, the lockdowns evoked a need to make contact with ourselves in a new way, opening us up to new possibilities.

The lockdowns also spawned accelerated creative outpourings in arts, humanities and sciences. A project at University College London, *Learning through Lockdown Dreams* saw MSc students examining dreams produced during the pandemic which were then discussed with psychoanalysts Daniel Pick and Liz Allison. At the same time, the British Artist David Downs created a series of sprawling images showing the virus' spores populating the sky, or, in another work, hundreds of hospital beds placed in a field so that this misplacing shocks us into recognising how many people have suffered and died, and the ghost-like effect this could have on those working in the UK's NHS and other health services. And science itself made huge leaps forward by developing a series of tests for the virus and then vaccines all produced at quite an extraordinary rate since necessity really had become the mother of invention.

Nevertheless, science alone was unable to address the ethical concerns thrown up by the pandemic. In John Wyndham's 1951 *The Day of the Triffids*, his languid British protagonist Bill Masen, reflecting on life before the collapse of society says:

> Looking back at the shape of things then, the amount we did not know and did not care to know about our daily lives is not only astonishing, but somehow a bit shocking' (p. 9).

Recent experience shows us that we have all lived day to day in varying degrees of unconsciousness of the inequalities, discrepancies, and artificial barriers and boundaries constructed in society and culture. Why have we been so divisive, so unaware, and, ironically, so isolationist? This is what can be studied so fruitfully now. But at the same time, it was easy to feel cross with those said to be in power who were apparently not doing enough, or who were making life unnecessarily difficult, or making decisions which to us seemed so obviously wrong. As Masen notes, 'It is humiliating to be dependant', and our dependency during lockdown accounts for much of the frustration many people experienced. But Masen then adds 'it's a still poorer pass to have no one to depend upon' (p. 4). Finding some level of gratitude that those responsible for our government and our care were able to act as rapidly and effectively as they did, in spite of errors and failures, is a more difficult achievement perhaps.

In this sense, the Covid19 pandemic robbed us of our autonomy and freedom, and made us dependent upon others in ways intensified by the knowledge that the decisions being made by others about us could have fatal consequence. One might say that it was a 'strange situation'. In Mary Ainsworth (1971) original 'strange situation' experiments in the 1970s, the children were placed under the mild stress of experiencing the withdrawal of their mothers just after a stranger had entered the room. This enabled the observers to notice and categorise a series of attachment patterns based on each child's response to this situation. The pandemic ruthlessly placed many of us in a similarly 'strange situation', a situation that mercilessly uncovered our underlying vulnerabilities and valencies. Firstly, our homes became all at once both our safe haven or secure base *and* our prison. The stranger who entered, and against which no door was secure, was the threat of illness and death by an invisible enemy. The parents in this case were the unreliable authorities and governments who, at times seemed to let us down, or were impotent to act effectively and keep us safe in this world. The notion that we could be kept entirely save at such a time however, could be seen as an idealising projection onto others, one which actually robs us of our own capacities and responsibility for protection.

Our relationship with social authorities may be based on and carry resonance of our earliest relationships with parental figures. This dynamic relationship with the official authorities and the effects that occur when it fails, is captured in Freudenburg's 1993, concept of 'recreancy'. Freudenburg derives the concept from ideas in Durkheim (1893). Recreancy is the 'failure to follow through on a duty or trust' (1993, p. 916) by a Government or other authority. In 2021 this was redefined in relation to the experience university students were having during COVID.19. The authors state that 'recreancy is loss of societal trust that results when institutional actors can no longer be counted on to perform their responsibilities' (p. 1), for example, governments and the university leadership teams. In this sense, there is a sudden loss in protection which is experienced as frightening. But what makes this worse is first, the shock felt in the realisation that we were unconscious of being protected, and second, that this protection was not secure. In fact, can it ever be felt as secure again? A way to reframe this in the terms of psychoanalysis would draw upon Freud's 1923 concept of the 'narcissistic injury'. In 'The infantile genital organisation: an interpolation into the theory of sexuality' (1923) Freud notes that 'a child gets the idea of a narcissistic injury through a bodily loss from the experience of losing his mother's breast after sucking' (p. 144). This reliable provision which is then rudely terminated (very like Winnicott's view of deprivation) is what causes the sense of injury and so this model grafts neatly onto the recognition of our profound vulnerability when governments and other social agents are seen and felt to fail, and their protection of us is withdrawn.

Using both sociological and psychoanalytic theorisations, the authors of this book track the way participants of their empirical study react and wrestle with the vicissitudes of their lockdown experience and how they managed the change, crisis and trauma that this evoked.

They describe the gradual social, political, economic and technological transformations that have occurred during the period of the pandemic, and which were accelerated because of it, including a distressing 'time disruption'. Drawing upon the trauma literature, they contrast these macro-changes with the micro-changes at the level of individual experience alluding to the 'disruption of continuity' (Nicholson, 2010) and the 'pandemic of poor mental health' that follows the physical pandemic. The trauma narrative here is not reductive, and draws upon psychosocial approaches that illustrate how opportunities for positive change and growth emerge, principally that of Papadopoulos' (2007) 'adversity activated development' which has made a substantial impact upon the literature and explores more hopeful and life-affirming responses to adverse experience.

The source material is a psychosocial reading of 46 interviews with Greek people living either in Athens, Greece or across 23 cities around the world. These semi-structured interviews were subjected to a psycho-analytically informed thematic analysis. A manifest strength here is that this is not a retrospective study but was conducted during the lockdown by two Greek researchers also immersed in their own reflexive experience. This gives the interviews an immediacy and impact that for readers of this book will be as stirring and evocative of their own experience as it certainly was for me. This engagement can lead to an internal dialogue and re-engagement with ones' own reactions and responses both, adaptive and problematic. Issues concerned with a lack of time-continuity, with isolation or symbiosis in relationships, with the struggle to maintain internal structure, the disorientation of loss and the mechanisms of denial and idealisation, or grief and mourning, used to accommodate it, are all observed. How participants narrate their experience of the 'crisis' differently suggests how broad and diverse the options were/are in terms of responses made to the same phenomena. Indeed, the authors noted in chapter one that the etymological root of the word 'crisis' means to 'choose, decide, and judge'. What determines reactions to crisis then is not the phenomena, or the traumatic events which everyone shared in common, but rather the internal world of subjectivity, which for each person is a unique configuration of dynamic forces and influences, ways of seeing and being which are based in the perception of experience and memory—that are always faulty and partial.

Social stratification is also tracked. The special concerns of Greek diaspora are noted—and one can see here a double isolation that comes with enforced isolation in a foreign land where contact with the familiarity of the motherland is withheld in a much more pronounced way. By contrast, the authors note (rather sadly) that the lockdown experience and the ensuing isolation may be so familiar to many elderly people that they don't experience this as a change. This is just one of the discrepancies and social inequalities mentioned above that emerges more clearly and vividly from this book.

The authors have created a fascinating exploration of how the pandemic has been experienced. They show the meaning-making process we go through under what may appear at first to be unique circumstances thrust upon us by firstly, hidden biological forces, but secondly, hidden psychical and social forces through which it is our human nature to respond. But in concluding this Foreword, I'm left thinking about the exceptional way in which we contextualise what has happened as a unique, once in a 100 years kind of event. Our strong human tendency is to anthropomorphise the world 'around us', and send, in our idealising fantasy, the sun around the earth, positioning ourselves in a privileged place of psychic retreat from the world as it is. But when the external world cannot be controlled, it is our internal capacities that we must turn to for both succour and adaptive resources. As we notice these 'black swans' with increasing frequency (the Russian invasion of Ukraine, and energy and cost of living crisis, the rise in the west of right wing political leadership) it seems pertinent that we should study ourselves under pressure. We must understand ourselves at both the social and psychic levels, and learn new and better ways to adapt and survive, ways that don't' fall into the groove of divisive paranoia or omnipotent fantasy. This book, and its exemplary authors, alongside all the interview participants, make a solid and timely contribution to this endeavour.

Chris Nicholson

References

Ainsworth, M. D. S., & Bell, S. M. (1970). Attachment, Exploration and Separation: Illustrated by the Behaviour of One-Year-Olds in a Strange Situation. *Child Development, 41*, 48–67.

Defeyter, M. A., Stretesky, P. B., Long, M. A., Furey, S., Reynolds, C., Porteous, D., Dodd, A,. Mann, E., Kemp A,. Fox, J., McAnallen, A., & Gonçalves, L. (2021). Mental Well-Being in UK Higher Education During Covid-19: Do Students Trust Universities and the Government? *Front. Public Health 9*, 646916. https://doi.org/10.3389/fpubh.2021.646916

Freud, S. (1923). The Infantile Genital Organisation: An Interpolation into the Theory of Sexuality. *Standard Edition, 19*, 141–145. London: Hogarth Press, 1961.

Freudenburg, W. R. (1993). Risk and Recreancy: Weber, the Division of Labor, and the Rationality of Risk Perceptions. *Soc For. 71*, 909–932. https://doi.org/10.2307/2580124

Pascal, B. (1987). *Pensées*. Middlesex: Penguin.

Wyndham, J. (1951). *The Day of the Triffids*. London: Penguin.

Acknowledgements

We would like to warmly thank the following colleagues and mentors for their unique contribution in this demanding as well as rewarding endeavour: a grateful thank you to Dr Chris Nicholson for his detailed guidance and enthusiastic support that enabled our arguments to become more clear and sharp. A huge thank you for Professor Kevin Featherstone's everlasting support all these years and particularly his encouragement and positive feedback. A more personal thank you to Dr Panagiotis Kostaras for his supportive insights and particularly enlightening and precise directions. Beyond our personalised acknowledgements, we would like to express our gratitude to the 46 participants who shared parts of their lives and souls during a very critical time of the Covid-19 pandemic.

Contents

List of Tables

1

Prolegomena

What does it mean to experience change, crisis and trauma while taking place simultaneously, in real time? How do we make sense of it? What does it mean and what does it feel like? How are we affected? Are we all affected in the same way, to the same extent?

Within the context of the Covid-19 pandemic, this book will explore the concepts of change, crisis and trauma as experienced, in real time, by 46 participants residing in 13 district countries and 23 cities around the world, during the April 2020 lockdowns. This book aims to answer the above questions by compressing them into just one: *What does this pandemic mean?*

In order for this question to be answered, more than one discipline had to be engaged in such endeavour, as such inquiry entails social as well as personal accounts. Exploring meaning-making, especially during the critical period of the first Covid-19 lockdown, requires analysis of real-time lived experiences of a rather challenging period on both personal and social levels. This study is the result of the synergy between sociological and psychosocial approaches in an attempt to describe, understand and explain how people have made meaning of this pandemic through their own lived experiences. This empirical exploration does not offer a retrospective account based on memory recalls of experienced lockdown; rather, it provides a live psychosocial study which took place during the first lockdown, when Covid-19 was at its height and making original and raw impact on participants.

Coronavirus bursts out as a global pandemic at the beginning of 2020 and soon became the ultimate determinant leading our personal, social and everyday lives during its ongoing duration. All humans have been affected to a greater or lesser degree; many of us have been infected, some of us have lost someone and perhaps all of us have suffered the consequences of this unique and rather awkward reality one way or the other. Different scientific disciplines have tried to contribute to the confrontation of this pandemic and certainly medical, pharmaceutical and all related research have been employed at the forefront. As time passed by, we started realising that the consequences of this pandemic have not been limited to causalities and health implications. The impact on mental health has been characterised as even greater than the impact on humans' health. Mental health had not been threatened by coronavirus itself, but rather through the desperate ways humans have followed in their attempt to protect themselves and their communities. Especially at the beginning of this pandemic's outburst when the 'unknown virus' had been spreading fear, uncertainty and even despair, while no one knew what was the best way to protect oneself from the threat of getting infected.

Various measures had been employed to protect against the spread of the pandemic. One of the first and the hardest had been the measure of lockdown entailing social distancing and isolation which had been followed by many, if not most, countries in different degrees, durations and periods of time.

Aims and Objectives

This book aims to explore whether meaning-making of the Covid-19 pandemic, and specifically during the period of the April 2020 lockdown, may derive from shared lived experiences among participants, who have gone through comparable circumstances simultaneously, albeit residing in diverse geographical regions. To accomplish this, we conducted 46 in-depth interviews with Greek participants (born and raised in Greece) residing in 13 district countries and 23 cities around the world.

The objective of the study is twofold: to reveal the meaning-making of the pandemic through the concepts of (a) change and crisis as well as (b) trauma and collective trauma. Regarding change and crisis, this book will offer a synthesised overview of this pandemic's meaning deriving from the lived experiences of the participants, which will be portrayed as a radical economic, political and social change, as well as a transformation of everyday life; as unsettlement and disruption of life continuity, as well as a fearful crisis but also one entailing the opportunity for improvement. In association with trauma and collective trauma, the pandemic will be further encountered as loss of space and time, loss of established ways of living, loss of time and life continuity as well as denial or acceptance of the loss of life prior to Covid-19.

This Study's Context

During the April 2020 lockdown the researchers found themselves in Athens. At that time nobody knew what the Covid-19 pandemic exactly was, how easily it could spread and what were the best measures to control it; there was no vaccine or cure, and people around the world were watching the numbers of infections and deaths rising progressively. At that point, Greece, like most countries, implemented the strictest measure of home isolation and limited unnecessary movement.

The first Covid-19 case in Greece was confirmed on 23 February 2020. Following most European countries, the Greek government at the time adopted a national lockdown (23 March–4 May), to delay the spread of coronavirus. The first lockdown (referred in this study as the April 2020 lockdown) included the following measures (also followed in most countries): (i) social isolation that restricts all but essential movement and economic activity, (ii) school and university closures, (iii) domestic travel restrictions, (iv) travel bans on visitors from high-risk countries and (v) quarantines for international visitors. The measures put in place in Greece had been among the most proactive and strictest in Europe. After a 42-day strict lockdown, Greece, like many other countries, began to gradually lift restrictions on movement and to restart business activity. Consequent lockdowns followed, and while most of the countries involved in this study followed similar measures at this time, the Greek government was one among the few that adopted more extreme policies.

The participants of this study reside in the following countries: Greece, Iceland, the UK, Belgium, Austria, Denmark, Germany, France, the Netherlands, the USA, Japan, Hong Kong and Bahrein. According to Oxford Coronavirus Government Response Tracker (OxCGRT, 2022) during April 2020 the measure of: "required to not leave the house with exceptions for daily exercise, grocery shopping, and 'essential' trips" has been implemented in the following countries: Greece, the UK, Belgium, Denmark, Austria, Germany, France, the Netherlands, the USA, Bahrain. Japan and China (including Hong Kong) followed the measure: "Recommended not to leave the house" whereas there are no reported measures for Iceland through this source. Thus, during the April 2020 lockdown, the 'stay at home' measure has been implemented in all of the countries where the participants of this study reside (with the exception of Iceland), and during the period of data collection (April 2020) all participants have been experienced comparable measures to a greater or lesser extent.

Rationale

During this lockdown, many people in Greece would seek permission through an SMS (sent to governmental authorities) to leave home for exercise purposes. Eirini Efsevia and I had long walks every evening, utilising the time we were allowed to spend away from home (within 2 km radius). During those walks we were talking about the consequences of the pandemic which reminded us rather vividly of the dramatic effects of the so-called Greek crisis which was supposedly completed recently (2008–2018).

It was during those walks that we started wondering whether Greeks may share similar understandings of what this pandemic means as we have all experienced adversity, especially due to the measure of social isolation. We, therefore, started piloting interviews exploring the ways Greeks have been experiencing the implementation of the protective measures taken by the Greek government and for that purpose we have initially collected 24 narrative interviews with adult Greek participants residing in Greece, mostly in Athens. Nonetheless, we shortly realised that our initial sample was rather restricted to regional limitations although we were studying a global phenomenon.

Although Greeks living within Greece share the commonality of shared socio-historical, cultural and regional realities, this pandemic may entail universal elements of meaning-making as the Covid-19 pandemic does not represent a national adversity, but rather, a global challenge. For example, Greeks living abroad have been experiencing lockdowns in different countries possibly in similar forms; might Greek diaspora perceive the meaning of this pandemic in a manner similar to Greeks living within Greece or not? Such realisation motivated the expansion of our study by including another 22 narrative interviews with Greeks permanently residing in 12 different countries around the globe, in an attempt to utilise an inclusive sample which maintains its national and socio-cultural characteristics but does not restrict itself regionally.

Enlarging our sample, in such an inclusive way, enabled this study to expand its regional limits in an attempt to explore whether the meaning-making of this pandemic might be collective among people who share common cultural experiences instead of regional similarities. And in order to maintain a national and socio-cultural coherence among participants, our access to the sizable, as well as global, Greek diaspora (Hellenism, 2022) offered an exceptional opportunity to include in our sample Greeks who live abroad and had been experiencing the Covid-19 pandemic through lockdowns, at the same time (April 2020) in different parts of the world. In this way, this study perceived those living in places other than Greece as a sort of 'control group' which enabled us to consider whether they experience lockdowns similarly to the country they are in, or alongside their Greek peers.

Why Change, Crisis and Trauma?

Considering and experiencing the period of the first quarantine and especially the measures of social isolation, the concepts of change, crisis and trauma were used more frequently than others during our discussions with Eirini Efsevia about the impact of the Covid-19 pandemic. We thus realised that we were unintentionally trying to find the most suitable terms able to depict the content and context of the emerging adversity. As the pandemic was a new reality for us (and everyone), we realised that characterising it solely as a tremendous change, or merely as a global crisis or purely as a collective traumatic experience, would result in a unilateral conceptualisation of this new reality. We therefore decided that we should join our epistemological forces and combine all three district, albeit, relevant concepts in our attempt to approach lived experiences of this pandemic as holistically as possible.

Synergies

This book has been written by two Greek female researchers affiliated to related but distinct disciplines. One is trained to conduct empirical research through sociological paradigms, whereas the other is trained to employ psychosocial and more specifically, psychoanalytic, approaches. This combination offered a fruitful synergy of two different approaches, as the first researcher has concentrated more on the impact of social circumstances upon lived experiences, whereas the second has focused on the ways individuals may process such lived experiences. By combining the different approaches, this study ultimately aims in contributing to a better understanding of the meaning-making of the Covid-19 pandemic through lived experiences of the April 2020 lockdowns.

An ideal way to study lived experiences derives from interpretive phenomenology as it brings to light what is taken for granted while allowing the emergence of phenomena from the perspective of how people interpret and attribute meaning to their existence; phenomenology, and more specifically hermeneutics, focuses on the interpretation of meaning through lived experience (Polit & Beck, 2012). As this study aims at exploring the meaning-making of Covid-19 lived experiences, interpretive phenomenology offers the ideal epistemological foundations in order to describe, understand and explain the meaning-making of Covid-19 through the ways participants have experienced the April 2020 lockdowns in different parts of the world.

Approaches

The theoretical approaches utilised in this study are rooted in two viewpoints:

(a) The *sociological* study of Covid-19 as social change, social crisis and its related consequences, incorporating current reviews of studies related to the impact of Covid-19 on various aspects of social and personal lives. Coping strategies have also been reviewed within the context of the pandemic.

(b) The *psychoanalytical* literature on trauma and particularly loss, including related psychosocial consequences, linked to studies on the impact of Covid-19 on mental health. Collective trauma has also been reviewed by incorporating a wider variety of theoretical approaches.

In terms of methods, qualitative data collection entailing 46 semi-structured in-depth interviews have been analysed according to thematic analysis rooted in both sociological and psychoanalytic theorisations. Analysis of data has utilised transcribed fragments of participants' lived experiences of April 2020 lockdowns, and has been divided into a sociological depiction of themes related to the wider concepts of change and crisis and a psychoanalytic illustration of themes associated with trauma and its consequences as well as collective trauma.

This book aims in offering an answer to the pressing question: What does this pandemic mean? To do so, this book employs a plurality of sociological and psychoanalytic approaches in order to identify, analyse, interpret and categorise the ways participants have experienced the Covid-19 pandemic. This book focuses on revealing the plurality of participants' emotions and the meaning ascribed to them associated with the impact of the pandemic on different aspects of life primarily associated with the themes of change, crisis and trauma.

Bibliography

Hellenism. (2022). Retrieved June 15, 2022, from https://hellenism.net/greece/greek-culture/greek-diaspora/

OxCGRT. (2022). Accessed June 15, 2022, from https://ourworldindata.org/covid-stay-home-restrictions#citation

Polit, D. F., & Beck, C. T. (2012). *Nursing Research: Generating and Assessing Evidence for Nursing Practice* (9th ed.). Lippincott Williams & Wilkins.

2

Social Change and Crisis

This chapter conceptualises the Covid-19 pandemic through the notions of social change and crisis. To do so, relevant definitions and theorisations for each concept have been employed and discussed against current literature on Covid-19. We argue that Covid-19 constitutes a social (as well as political, economic and historical) change which has been approached through its radical as well as gradual transformations effecting both macro and microsystems. Those transformations have been of such magnitude that this pandemic has also been depicted in terms of a global crisis which has disrupted continuity in various ways on both personal and social levels causing fearful frustration albeit also offering hopeful opportunities. Despite the fatal aftermath of this global crisis, most people have managed to survive it and some of them have even managed to excel through it.

Covid-19 Pandemic as Social Change

Social change can be described as the process of alteration(s) of certain social characteristics such as social structures and institutions, norms, values, cultural products and symbols (Calhoun, 1992). Silbereisen (2005) classifies change as (a) sudden/radical as it may occur quickly and

---

unexpectedly, for example, in the breakdown of the Soviet Union, a war, a natural disaster (and certainly an epidemic), characterised by a sudden revolution or transformation of all sectors of society, including the economic, social, political and legal systems; (b) gradual, which may last longer, as in the case of the demographic changes in many countries. The Covid-19 pandemic caused serious destructive consequential effects worldwide, particularly in deaths and economic burdens resulting in inevitable social transformations. These were due to the implementation of travel restrictions, social isolation, stay-at-home orders and quarantines adopted to curb the spread of the virus and minimise harm (Goh et al., 2020). In the light of such depiction, it might be easy to conclude that the Covid-19 pandemic falls into the first category of sudden/radical social change, as it emerged unexpectedly and expanded quickly within a limited period of time, altering reality in substantial ways, challenging health, economic, political and social systems. However, as we do not know yet the duration of the impacts of this global crisis, we cannot dismiss the prospect that this crisis actually entails gradual and perhaps less noticeable, albeit, non-reversible social transformations.

Perhaps the first attempt to systematically study social change and transformation derives from Durkheim's (1933/1893) study *Division of Labour in Society* which focuses on the shift from mechanistic to organic solidarity that in its extreme, leading to anomie. The state of anomie in a society creates feelings of discontent, meaninglessness, hopelessness and a sense of injustice: "The limits are unknown between the possible and the impossible, what is just and what is unjust, legitimate claims and hopes and those which are immoderate" (Durkheim, 1951/1897, p. 253). Such portrayal of social change would be associated with a rather radical form of social change and in such cases, employment is often affected early on in the form of loss of employment or through new requirements for flexibility, mobility and working with new technologies that may be required (Sennett, 1998). The Covid-19 pandemic entailed characteristic elements of radical social change as, for example, massive loss of employment (initially partial and gradual and eventually permanent) caused economic pressure, injury and illness (Goh et al., 2020) resulting in increased vulnerabilities especially regarding mental health (Brooks et al., 2020).

Radical social changes have an impact on all aspects of human life, such as education, employment, family life and even leisure (Sennett, 1998). Serious psychological repercussions have been reported caused by the wider unsettlement which has followed the pandemic and particularly because of the pandemic's social isolation periods, entailing fear, frustration and boredom which have been associated with post-traumatic symptoms, anxiety and depression (Brooks et al., 2020). Such description of unsettlement is clearly related to the state of 'anomie' which Durkheim coined in order to describe the aftermath of radical social transformations. Silbereisen et al. (2006) maintain that even once the initial period of rapid social change has been completed, individuals may still struggle to deal with the remaining aspects of social change such as the transformation of the economic system, and changes in family structure. Pratt (2020) maintains that the unfamiliarity of 'lockdown' has been a challenge to our societies and the ways we care for others; families, individuals and social groups have had to develop coping strategies of caring and schooling and employ creative combinations of demanding roles within the context of isolation.

Nevertheless, social transformation can also take place more slowly and gradually. Even in cases where social change has been associated with the concept of 'crisis', it has also been perceived as part of a standardised reality as 'crisis' demonstrates the ongoing novelty of our epoch, still perceived as a transition which ultimately leads to social change (Koselleck & Richter, 2006). Similarly, social change even in the forms of globalisation, individualisation and pluralisation of biographical trajectories, as well as demographic change, is perceived as gradual transformation which has led to an increase in uncertainty in people's lives in a number of different domains (Pinquart & Silbereisen, 2004). Indeed, social transformations are part of our everyday lives and quite often take place without necessarily realising it, for example, the social impact of technological evolution, climate change and economic crisis, the results of global movements like 'me too' and 'black lives matter' (Alexander, 2012). Such gradual transformations though may have enabled more permanent alterations to take place because of the pandemic.

May (2011) perceives social change as the ongoing alteration in the dynamic of societies as people and relations change. Social change and the endless forms of interactions are constantly interrelated and both affecting each other. Change tends to be constant and incremental and is introduced gradually into our lives in the form of, for example, new technologies, new institutional practices, new forms of 'culture' and the changing requirements of the workplace. Ultimately, people's reaction to much of social change forms gradual alterations in (some aspect of) their habits, routines and ways of thinking and in that way, people contribute to further social transformations. Such gradual shifts have been evident before the pandemic whereas they have been intensified during the pandemic as the ongoing technological evolution has now been transformed to a universal everyday reality during and because of the pandemic. Screen time substituting leisure activities has increased during the pandemic, with excessive use of social media and online gaming. The use of online learning has created a new reality also utilised in all levels of education (Oosterhoff et al., 2020) resulting in increased reliance on digital technologies to enable some continuity of social and working lives (Pratt, 2020). Therefore, the gradual technological advancement was ultimately utilised and adopted as people globally heavily relied on it, in order to complete employment, education and leisure activities on a daily basis.

It is thus understood, that in the case of the Covid-19 pandemic, we refer to a process of social change entailing elements of radical as well as gradual social, political and economic transformations. In order to cope with such plurality and magnitude of alterations, people needed to adjust and, in most cases, alter their everyday lives accordingly. Silbereisen and Eye (1999) explain that, historically, individuals and groups of individuals have always subjected themselves and were subjected by others to situations where adaptation to change and transitions was a necessity. The authors distinguish between forceful change (including slavery, expulsion or dislocation) and voluntary change (involving movement of individuals like migration). However, radical political and social changes involve different characteristics as the need for adaptation to change can be felt by everybody and refers to a change that came to the people; there was no journey needed nor relocation. The change arrives suddenly and all individuals have to deal with it.

The Covid-19 pandemic is reflected in the description of such radical social and political changes as people universally had to adapt urgently to a new reality without having to be relocated or dislocated and certainly without being prepared. Examples of universal lifestyle changes include replacement of in-person schooling with virtual education, loss of social interaction with teachers, friends and peers, cessation of extra-curricular activities, and virtual graduation replacing in-person ceremonies (Cardenas et al., 2020). Consequently, the Covid-19 pandemic can be perceived as social change that has taken place radically and rapidly but at the same time is still ongoing, as it also entails elements of gradual social, political, economic and even technological transformations. The ways people adjust to the new realities may determine not only the ways Covid-19 has been perceived but also experienced as social change.

This section approached the Covid-19 pandemic through the concept of social change, by critically discussing some of the latest sociological studies on the Covid-19 pandemic against definitions and conceptualisations of radical and gradual social change. It has been argued that the Covid-19 pandemic entails a plurality of conceptualisations ascribed to the notion of social change primarily associated with its radical, disruptive and sudden impacts of the ways societies operate and people live their lives. At the same time, the Covid-19 pandemic entails elements of gradual social change as the Covid-19 pandemic allowed the intensification of pre-existing technological interventions which are currently and gradually shaping new forms of everyday living. The following section attempts to identify the ways Covid-19 (as social change) affects the way people live their lives.

The Effect of Covid-19 as Social Change

Even in the case of radical crisis, social change does not affect all individuals in the same way. Pinquart and Silbereisen (2004) explain that the impact of social change on each person can be perceived through two systems: (a) the macrosystem, referring to transformations in society through changing laws or political and social institutions, and by new access to technical innovations; (b) microsystems, referring to the ways individuals relate to one another through alterations in family, school, or workplace, which in turn affect the individual itself. The authors maintain that most of the effects of social change on the level of society are mediated through the microsystems. As a result of the Covid-19 pandemic, governments around the world have implemented various methods of social restrictions in an attempt to reduce transmission (Harris et al., 2021); such measures causing significant alterations in everyday life can be perceived as the alterations in the macrosystem. In terms of the microsystem and how the Covid-19 pandemic has affected the ways people interact with one another, Covid-19 had a tremendous impact on mental health on both personal and collective levels (Cardenas et al., 2020).

The impact of social change on macrosystems can also be seen when political violence is so substantial that the elements that shape community life (e.g. norms, spaces, and practices) have been systematically destroyed or transformed, collective memories, social experiences and practices may be completely different from one generation to another (Spini et al., 2014). Individual agency can therefore be limited due to historical events beyond individual control, such as changes in the labour market, economic downturns or discrete historical events such as the outbreak of war (Elder, 1974/1999). There is a close relationship between individual development and societal progress (Silbereisen, 2005). In the case of the Covid-19 pandemic, the aftermath is still ongoing, but in terms of social consequences, Grasso et al. (2020) have categorised the impact of the Covid-19 crisis on European societies as follows: (a) social inequalities (gender inequalities, ethnicity and otherness, education, labour market); (b) solidarity and cohesion—which could be threatened but also strengthened in those cases that collective trauma reinforces social trust relations (Alexander 2012); (c) governance and welfare state; (d) psychological aspects (well-being and resilience vs stress and anxiety); and (e) culture and lifestyles.

Grasso et al. (2020) maintain that the Covid-19 crisis can be seen as a catalyst, speeding up some social processes and bringing others close in relation to social tension and divisions, inequalities and power imbalances, but also revealing the capacity for collective problem-solving and solidarity among people and societies. The United Nations (2021) has identified three main determinants of Covid-19 strategies that have allowed specific countries to perform relatively well in coping with the pandemic: healthcare, social protection and overall governance systems

(United Nations, 2021); consequently, these are the main areas in which improvement needs to be reinforced.

Different cultures share different understandings about the level of tolerance between areas of thinking and behaving and therefore, psychological consequences of social change depend upon the intensity of social pressure to change old behaviours (Pinquart & Silbereisen, 2004). For example, the study of Zhou et al. (2020) revealed mental health consequences of the Covid-19 pandemic in China, involving excessive worrying, irritability, home confinement and fear of infection and transmission which are associated with mild to severe anxiety symptoms during the pandemic.

At the same time, transitions enable or even force individuals to negotiate their own life, involving opportunities as well as constraints for individual agency. In those cases, we focus on the impact of social change on microsystems. Social change determines the form of transition, impacting on the timing or the sequencing of events. The way individuals attempt to cope with social transformation can be linked with historical time, as individual lives are mutually shaped by personal characteristics and the socio-historical context. Therefore, negotiating transitions depends upon the differences in individuals, the timing of social change and the wider socio-historical context in which the transition occurs (Schoon, 2007). In the case of the Covid-19 pandemic, the meaning of the socio-historical context might have become vague, as unprecedented, universal measures have been implemented beyond the socio-historical context of specific regions. Indicatively, the distinct measure of self-isolation during lockdowns has formed a rather unique "disruption of continuity" (Nicholson, 2010) during the Covid-19 pandemic affecting personal as well as social life. According to the relevant literature, isolation could be a risk factor for deterioration in mental health, including depressive and anxiety symptoms, distress, fear, post-traumatic stress and insomnia.

The global context of this pandemic allowed a unique kind of phobia to emerge, termed by some scholars "Covid-19 Phobia" (Lindinger-Sternart et al., 2021) and by others "Coronaphobia" (Asmundson & Taylor, 2020; Brooks et al., 2020), referring to anxiety disorders resulting from the fear of Covid-19. "Coronaphobia" has enhanced anxiety symptoms, with a further aggravating role mediated by isolation at home (Brooks et al., 2020). The impact of the lockdown measures, in particular, includes loss of freedom, interruption of daily routines (Bao et al., 2020; Duan & Zhu, 2020) and the elimination of social contacts (Best et al., 2020) leading to personal and social uncertainties, loss of control and increased psychological disorders (Brooks et al., 2020). The consequences of April 2020 (and consequent) lockdowns related to sense of isolation fear, uncertainty (Gori & Topino, 2021; Ren et al., 2020; Wang et al., 2020), loneliness, psycho-social distress and lower levels of life-satisfaction (Benke et al., 2020). In fact the impact of the pandemic (and particularly lockdowns), in terms of social change on microsystems along with the way people have related to each other during this, has been of such magnitude and consequence that some experts have used the term "parallel mental health pandemic" (Cardenas et al., 2020). Alongside the immediate physical health effects of the Covid-19, a secondary mental health pandemic is seen to follow.

Consequently, approaching the Covid-19 pandemic as a social change enables us to realise that the effect of its radical as well as gradual transformations can be experienced through macro and microsystems as the pandemic has caused definite alterations on both social and personal levels. The magnitude of such social change that Covid-19 entails has also been captured in terms of 'crisis' in an attempt to grasp the extent of the effect caused on people's lives.

Covid-19 Pandemic as Crisis

The French, German and English words *la crise* ('the crisis'), *die Krise* ('the crisis') and 'crisis' have the common Greek root originating from the verb 'krino', which means choose, decide and judge, and this implies that events of a certain magnitude force such choosing, deciding and judging upon us. The idea of crisis has been connected with danger that was supposed to coexist with fear (Koselleck & Richter, 2006). Crisis is one of the terms repeatedly used to describe Covid-19 in everyday language. Ward (2020) explains that there are specific sociological concepts involved in the study of the Covid-19 pandemic, one of which is 'crisis', and more specifically, Fuchs (2020) uses the term "corona crisis" to describe the fact that social reality has been interrupted and altered during the pandemic whereas routines and everyday practices were completely reorganised. The meaning of crisis has been connected with the danger which is supposed to coexist with fear and uncertainty (Tangjia, 2014). Fear and panic have certainly been fundamental components of the pandemic which has been reported as "Covid-19 phobia" (Lindinger-Sternart et al., 2021) and "Coronaphobia" (Asmundson & Taylor, 2020; Brooks et al., 2020); fear has also been generated by media especially in relation to economic global disaster(s) (Monaghan, 2020) and, characteristically, Žižek (2020, p. 85) warned that an "economic mega-crisis is likely". Additional forms of fear relate to the elimination of human freedom (Caduff, 2020), exaggerated public health measures (Brown, 2020) and concerns have been raised about a "pedagogy of fear" (Monaghan, 2020). Crisis has been perceived as a dangerous state of affairs that becomes a threat to continuity and stability and may lead to fatal results. In fact, humans are either defeated in the crisis, survive or become its victim (Tangjia, 2014), while, according to Strong (1990, p. 249), major outbreak of novel, fatal epidemic disease can quickly be followed by both plagues of fear, panic, suspicion and stigma. The way people will collectively react to pandemics ultimately relates with the ways people interact. Within this context Möhring et al. (2020) revealed a number of stressors associated to Covid-19 pandemic in Germany like: economic hardship, job loss, increased health risks and uncertainties, a reduction of social contacts outside of the household, increased screen time and fewer opportunities for physical activity.

Hall (2019) provides perhaps the most concrete and topical depiction of the concept of crisis and clearly associates the concept with that of change and unsettlement: "Crises are characterised by a jarring or disruption of time, momentum, and change: the fracturing, fragility, rupturing, and instability of the current, or an anticipated, situation. The time over which crises occur, and their pace, is nevertheless marked into lived/social time, taking place in 'real time'" (Hall, 2019, p. 479). Such depiction can capture the magnitude, impact and depth of the Covid-19 pandemic as it reflects the outrageous global disruption of time and continuity along with collective feelings of uncertainty and vulnerability among humans experienced on a universal level. Ward (2020) explains that Covid-19 is primarily related to concepts of risk, fear, panic and trust (or lack of) as well as individualisation, isolation, stigma, globalisation and uncertainty.

Lately, the idea of crisis is also associated with climate change, financial volatility, biodiversity loss, food insecurity, rampant labour-market informalisation and so on. Crisis has been perceived as a process through which new ways of ordering the relations between humans and the rest of nature take shape (Moore, 2017). For Tangjia, it partly originates from the greediness of human nature and affects peoples' emotions, ways of thinking and acting, while the globalisation of the economy leads to globalisation of these crises, including the rapid spreading of viruses (e.g. HIV/AIDS) which has become a symbol of the globalisation of diseases (Tangjia, 2014). The Covid-19 pandemic portrays exactly such a globalised crisis as it does not only threaten each and everyone's health but has caused an enormous economic catastrophe leading to altered ways of living (Nicola et al., 2020). The pandemic can also be perceived through Meszaros' (2014) term of "structural crisis" as referring to the cases that the totality of a social complex is affected including all its relations with its constituent parts or subcomplexes, as well as with other complexes to which it is linked. A structural crisis ultimately questions the very existence of the overall complex concerned (in the case of Covid-19, global health, social and economic spheres), leading to the replacement by some alternative complex; thus, it is concerned with the ultimate limits of a global structure. Indicative reactions to the Covid-19 pandemic were a questioning of overall structures. This became especially apparent through the form of distrust towards governments, statistics, science, media, technology (Calnan, 2020), political institutions (Risi et al., 2020) and even other people (Ward, 2020), whereas Monaghan (2020, p. 1989) adds the reactions of "frustration, anger, disbelief, resignation, boredom, disappointment and disdain towards authorities acting in a draconian and inconsistent manner".

At the same time, according to Tangjia (2014), crisis can offer self-immunisation to society and provide possibilities for improvement and development as it stimulates social systems to protect themselves by recognising their own vulnerability to disease but also by looking for ways to overcome it. This pattern can be seen clearly through the current pandemic especially if we consider that, as Meszaros (2014) maintains, crisis might be controllable at its initial stage, but as time proceeds, the destructive force becomes stronger and, without intervention, it proliferates very quickly. Such a realisation becomes evident once we consider the consequences of Covid-19, beyond fatalities. It has been widely acknowledged that during this pandemic the elderly are predominantly suffering coronavirus' physical consequences whereas youth are suffering the social impacts of lockdowns (Matthewman & Huppatz, 2020). People of colour have been particularly effected due to socio-economic volubility whereas women specifically have been globally affected more as they form the larger part of health and social-care professions (Boniol et al., 2019); they still offer the largest part of unpaid work (Battyany, 2020), and they have been the main ones to combine housework, childcare and work-from-home activities (Collins et al. 2020; Möhring et al., 2020; Risi et al., 2020). Concerns about mental health implications for all age groups have been repeatedly raised (Monaghan, 2020). Tangjia (2014) emphasises that crisis exposes the symptoms of society, particularly serious but hidden social problems continuing in the name of prosperity. In the case of Covid-19 such symptoms were primarily related with racism, inequalities, violent attacks (WHO, 2021), as well as stigma and xenophobia as people travelling during the pandemic are the ones "spreading the virus" and thus immigrants are placed in the spotlight (Ward, 2020).

Notably, the psycho-social significance and relevance of the study of (any) crisis and its meaning relates with the way crisis may be involved in the shaping and reshaping of subjectivity as it is lived and challenged through the emergence of new social practices and social struggles (Meszaros, 2014). For example, the extended periods people had to remain in their homes during the pandemic in Germany resulted in a general, pronounced decrease in family satisfaction as well as parenthood (Möhring et al., 2020). Whereas for those without children, the negative lockdown effect may result from the elimination of social contacts (Best et al. 2020). Risi et al. (2020) explained that during the Covid-19 pandemic in Italy, the emergent lack of personal spaces, the complex management of different social roles and the collapse of the traditional boundaries between professional and private life resulted in a stress overload.

Following the depiction of Covid-19 as a radical as well as gradual social change affecting both macro and microsystems, this section approached this pandemic through the concept of crisis, by critically discussing some of the latest sociological studies on the Covid-19 pandemic utilising sociological definitions and conceptualisations of crisis. It becomes understandable that this pandemic entails a plurality of conceptualisations ascribed to the notion of crisis primarily associated with its negative, fearful and disruptive meaning-making at the structural level and saw conflictual social dynamics and negative impacts on the ways people live their lives. The following section focuses on the effects of Covid-19 as crisis especially on the ways people live their lives at the social level, while finding opportunities for new understandings and co-operations.

The Effect of Covid-19 as Crisis

Dinerstein et al. (2014) explain that researchers need to focus on the study of the ways in which the crisis can generate existential problems (often related to anxiety and depression) in order to understand the impact of crisis on subjectivity. Although we tend to find the reasons for crisis outside ourselves, self-reflection enables us to evaluate ourselves in relation to our social context and become able to recognise our capacities and limitations. The ways each one of us is related to others during crisis can be successfully established once we are in sympathy with the situation of others also in crisis. Through the feelings of sympathy and empathy towards others, we are able to realise that we are part of the same situation, community and destiny (Tangjia, 2014). Lived experiences of crises ultimately become manifestations of life crisis shaping life course, biographies and imaginaries of the future. In that sense, economic, political or social crises convert to personal crises (Hall, 2019). Regarding the Covid-19 pandemic, Monbiot (2020) notes the rise of volunteering among young people, offering support in various contexts, and this is further supported by Lourens (2020) who refers to the lessons people have learned about "being in this together" during the crisis.

French et al. (2009, p. 2549) add that "crises are about change ... [and] opportunities to impose new ideas and practices". Crisis can also be shared, relational, diverging and intersecting with the conjunctures of others, for example, within family, generation or community; crisis can become part of the everyday, as well as future imaginaries, manifesting as a very personal crisis (Hall, 2019). Tangjia maintains that as crisis can determine the ways people live their lives, it can reveal each person's capacity, courage and wisdom and helps us adjust ourselves to new situations and to understand ourselves in new ways despite causing dramatic change to living conditions and human relationships. Therefore, crisis does not only cause worry and fear but also anticipation and hope (Tangjia, 2014) as it can offer possibilities for change and continuity while forming lived, intimate and very personal experiences (Hall, 2019).

Matthewman and Huppatz (2020) explain that disasters, like the Covid-19 pandemic, are essentially social phenomena and consequent threats and experiences are public and shared. Collective adversity may create social solidarity providing the basis for physical and emotional support. They remind us that humans are social beings and thus products of culture and collective labour; they can be remarkably altruistic, resilient and generous, committed to the possibility of doing things differently, desiring of human connection and purpose. In disasters, then, people may experience different social energies, including altruism and caring, resulting in new self-definitions like being for others not only for ourselves. This pandemic revealed the remarkable altruism of people as well as new kinds of power-dynamics (in terms of who and what counts) and the belief that alternative ways of living are possible (Matthewman & Huppatz, 2020, pp. 5–6). Thus, Covid-19 perceived as crisis does not only entail fearful and negative connotations. Rather positive and hopeful approaches have also been ascribed as a consequence of such radical social change depicted as a global crisis.

So far, the Covid-19 pandemic has been discussed as a radical as well as gradual change, causing transformations to both micro and macrosystems resulting in a global crisis which entails fearful as well as hopeful connotations. Crises of such magnitude and intensity, having resulted in such sudden and even irreversible transformations, inevitably make us wonder how people have been able to cope with it. The following section begins to consider by engaging with some of the relevant literature.

Coping Strategies

Life-course research (Elder, 1999/1974) strongly emphasises the individual experience of collective threats, such as economic crises or wars, and it informs us that there is significant variability in the way major historical traumas, such as the Great Depression of the 1930s or World War II, were experienced. As will be further discussed in the next chapter, different people experience traumatic events in distinct ways (Papadopoulos, 2007), whereas collective trauma may not be the result of collective pain (Alexander, 2012). The fact that traumatic experiences may be shared is an important factor in mitigating distress and anxiety that these events create (Kearns et al., 2017). A sense of shared experience can contribute to feelings of collective efficacy which in turn is likely to contribute to psychological resilience. Home (2020) and Neal (1998) add that in cases where disruptive events occur, new opportunities for innovation and change may also emerge. Therefore, crises and radical social change does not only cause worry and fear but also anticipation and hope (Tangjia, 2014) as they can offer possibilities for change and continuity while forming lived, intimate and very personal experiences (Hall, 2019). Perhaps it is for these reasons that Bacevic and McGoey (2021) maintain that during the Covid-19 pandemic peoples' capacity for adaption, reflection and social organisation has been evident.

Some people are more vulnerable to social change, in case they have to face changes unprecedented in their prior life and thus being unprepared to confront them. However, if change is closer to their previous lives and they have already developed coping mechanisms, then exposure to stress is manageable (Rutter, 1994). However, social change that does not allow individuals to maintain effectively habitual behaviours results in a sense of loss of control over one's life (Silbereisen, 2005). The literature suggests that during the pandemic social support, positive lifestyle behaviours, social media used for the purpose of maintaining social contact, and even mindfulness, have been some of the main coping strategies utilised in particularly stressful settings like those experienced by medical professionals (Bohlken et al., 2020; Du et al., 2020). Reduced exposure to negative media content during the pandemic has also been noted as a helpful coping strategy (Guo et al., 2020).

Papadopoulos claims that there are people who not only survive challenging circumstances but also become strengthened by the particular exposure to adversity. This response is termed "Adversity Activated Development" (Papadopoulos, 2004, 2006) and refers to the positive developments that are a direct result of being exposed to adversity. It is possible that people may find meaning in their suffering and can transform their negative experience in a positive way, giving meaning to suffering that can be transformative (Frankl, 1959). Studies of psycho-social resilience had attempted to explain how people living in a difficult world can prioritise positivity and hope (Bartley, 2006; Ungar, 2004). Resilience is particularly relevant to the context of Covid-19 as, according to Masten, it relates to "phenomena characterized by good outcomes in spite of serious threats to adaptation or development" (Masten, 2001, p. 228). In fact Lindinger-Sternart et al. (2021) suggest that resilience can be a protective factor against mental health problems that are related to adverse experiences like the Covid-19 pandemic. According to their study, the highest level of resilience towards Covid-19 phobia was found among American participants, followed by Europeans, Pakistanis, Indians and Indonesians. The findings of this study also suggest that the higher the age of participants, the higher the level of resilience towards Covid-19 phobia, which suggests that experience of prior adversity may be adaptive.

Resilience may also be perceived in terms of 'coping mechanisms' or adaptation to new social, economic and political situations. In challenging times people may re-adjust claims and resources or may develop new ways of behaving in order to meet the new challenges. A new equilibrium is achieved when claims match resources (Silbereisen & Chen, 2010; Elder & Caspi, 1990). Pinquart and Silbereisen (2004) add that resource-rich individuals are expected to show active, problem-focused coping and adaptive abilities resulting from radical social alterations, be prepared to overcome adverse circumstances and be able to take advantage of emerging new opportunities. Coping strategies that have proven helpful during the pandemic have been identified by researchers and include seeking social support, positive thinking, and problem-solving should be encouraged, with the positive role of the media being fundamental in this respect (Anwar, et al., 2020). At the same time, younger people and particularly children have developed distinct ways of coping with the pandemic.

Coping strategies that children have utilised in order to cope with the adversity they have experienced include seeking social support via social media and searching for distraction; interestingly, it was helpful for older children to search for Covid-19-related information whereas for younger children avoiding news media has helped them to better regulate their emotions (Cauberghe et al., 2021).

The more uncertain and undefined new challenges are, the more likely it is that old, albeit, successful behavioural strategies will be used (Elder & Caspi, 1990). Self-efficacy has been identified as an important resource in mastering rapid change of social and political systems. As social change is often revealed and experienced as unpredictable and undermining, a hopeful way to support more productive negotiations of new challenges is by empowering people through strengthening individual and social resources prior to the emergence of the transitional period. Such support could focus on the areas of self-efficacy, planning competence and educational attainment (Pinquart & Silbereisen, 2004). For example, studies on the impact of the Covid-19 pandemic on students emphasise the significance of utilisation of social networks, the effectiveness of empathetic communication system and the helpfulness of adaptive expression and emotional management (Morales-Rodríguez, 2021) that educational institutions could have set in place as supportive mechanisms in times of crisis or radical change.

Tangjia (2014) maintains that although crisis often appears suddenly and people do not have enough time to react and take action, we can nevertheless work out some plans to cope with crisis ahead of time by putting positive and useful elements into full use to eliminate crisis. In this vein, the United Nations emphasises the necessity of the immediate establishment of a universal healthcare and social protection system along with improving governance even by developing countries (United Nations, 2021). Such proactive protective measures may prevent future re-occurrences of the current disastrous effects of the pandemic, or may better control and minimise the damage, caused in each case.

The Covid-19 pandemic has been portrayed as an unprecedented global crisis causing colossal social, political and economic transformations experienced traumatically, to a greater or lesser extent; still, despite its disastrous and lethal aftermath, most people have survived it and, in doing so, coping strategies have been employed. This section focused on the more hopeful perception of the pandemic, despite its primary depiction as a crisis entailing inevitable social alterations as well as traumatic components. This pandemic has also been depicted as an opportunity for positive change, development and progress.

Synopsis

This chapter has provided a brief and a theoretical overview of the Covid-19 pandemic through the concepts of social change and crisis. We have argued that Covid-19 constitutes a social (as well as political, economic and historical) change which has been approached through its radical as well as gradual transformations effecting both the macro and microsystems. Those transformations have been of such magnitude that this pandemic has also been depicted in terms of a global crisis which has disrupted continuity in various ways on both personal and social levels causing fearful frustration albeit also offering hopeful opportunities. Nevertheless, despite the fatal aftermath of such a traumatic crisis, most people have managed to survive it and some of them have even managed to grow or excel through it.

The following chapter will expand on the experiences of Covid-19 by exploring this through the concept of trauma, entailing elements of personal and collective trauma especially associated with the essence of loss, deriving primarily from psychoanalytic perspectives.

Bibliography

Alexander, J. (2012). *Trauma: a Social Theory*. Polity.

Anwar, A., Malik, M., Raees, V., & Anwar, A. (2020). Role of Mass Media and Public Health Communications in the COVID-19 Pandemic. *Cureus, 12*, e10453–e10453.

Asmundson, G. J. G., & Taylor, S. (2020). Coronaphobia: Fear of the 2019-nCoV Outbreak. *Journal of Anxiety Disorders, 70*, 102196.

Bacevic, J., & McGoey, L. (2021). *Surfing Ignorance: Covid-19 And The Rise Of Fatalistic Liberalism, Research Repository.* University of Essex (Unpublished). http://repository.essex.ac.uk/30721/

Bao, Y., Sun, Y., Meng, S., Shi, J., & Lu, L. (2020). 2019-nCoV epidemic: Address Mental Health Care to Empower Society. *Lancet, 395*(10224), e37–e38.

Bartley, M. (2006). *Capability and Resilience: Beating the Odds.* University College London, Department of Epidemiology and Public Health.

Battyany, K. (2020). The Covid-19 Pandemic Reveals and Exacerbates the Crisis of Care. *Open Democracy.* https://www.opendemocracy.net/en/openmovements/covid-19-pandemic-reveals-and-exacerbates-crisis-care/

Benke, C., Autenrieth, L. K., Asselmann, E., & Pané-Farré, C. A. (2020). Lockdown, Quarantine Measures, and Social Distancing: Associations with Depression, Anxiety and Distress at the Beginning of the COVID-19 Pandemic Among Adults from Germany. *Psychiatry Research, 293*, 113462.

Best, L. A., Law, M. A., Roach, S., & Wilbiks, J. M. P. (2020). The Psychological Impact of COVID-19 in Canada: Effects of Social Isolation During the Initial Response. *Canadian Psychology.* Advance online publication. https://doi.org/10.1037/cap0000254

Bohlken, J., Schömig, F., Lemke, M. R., Pumberger, M., & Riedel-Heller, S. G. (2020). COVID-19 Pandemic: Stress Experience of Healthcare Workers: A Short Current Review. *Psychiatrische Praxis, 47*, 190–197.

Boniol, M., McIsaac, M., Xu, L., Wuliji, T., Diallo, K., & Campbell, J. (2019). *Gender Equity in the Health Workforce: Analysis of 104 Countries.* Geneva: World Health Organization. https://apps.who.int/iris/bitstream/handle/10665/311314/WHOHIS-HWF-Gender-WP1-2019.1-eng.pdf

Brooks, S. K., Webster, R. K., Smith, L. E., Woodland, L., Wessely, S., Greenberg, N., & Rubin, G. J. (2020). The Psychological Impact of Quarantine and How to Reduce it: Rapid Review of the Evidence. *Lancet, 395*(10227), 912–920.

Brown, R. D. (2020). Public Health Lessons Learned from Biases in Coronavirus Mortality Overestimation. *Disaster Medicine and Public Health Preparedness, 14*, 1–24.

Caduff, C. (2020). What Went Wrong: Corona and the World after the Full Stop. *Medical Anthropology Quarterly, 34*(4), 467–487.

Calhoun, C. (1992). Social Change. In E. F. Borgatta & M. L. Borgatta (Eds.), *Encyclopedia of Sociology* (Vol. 4, pp. 1807–1812). Macmillan.

Calnan, M. (2020). Health Policy and Controlling Covid-19 in England: Sociological Insights. *Emerald Open Research, 2*(40), 2–14. https://doi.org/10.35241/emeraldopenres.13726.2

Cardenas, M. C., Bustos, S. S., & Chakraborty, R. (2020). A 'parallel pandemic': The Psychosocial Burden of COVID-19 in Children and Adolescents. *Acta Pædiatrica, 109*(11), 2187–2188.

Cauberghe, V., De Jans, S., Hudders, L., & Vanwesenbeeck, I. (2021). Children's Resilience during Covid-19 confinement. A Child's Perspective–Which General and Media Coping Strategies are Useful? *Journal of Community Psychology, 50*, 1–18.

Collins, C., Landivar, L. C., Ruppanner, L., & Scarborough, W. J. (2020). COVID-19 and the Gender Gap in Work Hours. *Gender, Work & Organization.* https://doi.org/10.1111/gwao.12506.

Dinerstein, A. C., Schwartz, G., & Taylor, G. (2014). Sociological Imagination as Social Critique: Interrogating the 'Global Economic Crisis. *Sociology, 48*(5), 859–868.

Du, J., Dong, L., Wang, T., Yuan, C., Rao, F., Zhang, L., Liu, B., Zhang, M., Yin, Y., Qin, J., Bouey, J., Zhao, M., & Li, X. (2020). Psychological Symptoms Among Frontline Healthcare Workers during COVID-19 Outbreak in Wuhan. *General Hospital Psychiatry, 67*, 144–145.

Duan, L., & Zhu, G. (2020). Psychological Interventions for People Affected by the COVID-19 Epidemic. *Lancet Psychiatry, 7*(4), 300–302.

Durkheim, E. (1933[1893]). *The Division of Labor in Society* (G. Simpson, Trans.). The Free Press.

Durkheim, E. (1951[1897]). *Suicide: A Study in Sociology* (J. A. Spaulding and G. Simpson, Trans.). The Free Press.

Elder, G. H. (1974/1999). *Children of the Great Depression: Social Change in life Experience.* Westview Press. [First published 1974].

Elder, G. H., Jr., & Caspi, A. (1990). Studying Lives in a Changing Society: Sociological and Personological Explorations. In A. I. Rabin, R. A. Zucker, R. A. Emmons, & S. Frank (Eds.), *Studying Persons and Lives* (pp. 201–247). Springer Publishing Co.

Frankl, V. (1959). *Man's Search for Meaning.* Washington Square Press.

French, S., Leyshon, A., & Thrift, N. (2009). A Very Geographical Crisis: The Making and Breaking of the 2007–2008 Financial Crisis. *Cambridge Journal of Regions, Economy and Society, 2*(2), 287–302.

Fuchs, C. (2020). 'Everyday life and everyday Communication in Coronavirus Capitalism', Triple C: Communication, Capitalism & Critique. *Open Access Journal for a Global Sustainable Information Society, 18*(1), 375–398.

Goh, K. K., Lu, M. L., & Jou, S. (2020). 'Impact of COVID-19 Pandemic: Social Distancing and the Vulnerability to Domestic Violence. *Psychiatry and Clinical Neurosciences', 74*(11), 612–613.

Gori, A., & Topino, E. (2021). Across the COVID-19 waves—Assessing Temporal fluctuations in Perceived Stress, Post-Traumatic Symptoms, Worry, Anxiety and Civic Moral Disengagement Over One Year of Pandemic. *International Journal of Environmental Research and Public Health, 18*(11), 5651.

Grasso, M., Klicperová-Baker, M., Koos, S., Kosyakova, Y., Petrillo, A., & Vlase, I. (2020). The Impact of the Coronavirus Crisis on European Societies., What Have We Learned and Where Do We Go From Here? Introduction to the Covid Volume. *European Societies., 23*(s1), 2–32.

Guo, J., Feng, X. L., Wang, X. H., & van I Jzendoorn, M. H. C. (2020). Coping with COVID-19: Exposure to COVID-19 and Negative Impact on Livelihood Predict Elevated Mental Health Problems in Chinese Adults. *International Journal of Environmental Research and Public Health, 17*, 3857.

Hall, S. M. (2019). A Very Personal Crisis: Family Fragilities and Everyday Conjunctures Within Lived Experiences of Austerity. *Transactions of the Institute of British Geographers, 44*, 479–492.

Harris, D., Ellis, D. Y., Gorman, D., Foo, N., & Haustead, D. (2021). Impact of COVID-19 Social Restrictions on Trauma Presentations in South Australia. *Emergency medicine Australasia, 33*(1), 152–154.

Home. (2020, July). Collective Trauma Amid Covid: Excerpt from 'Together Apart'. https://www.socialsciencespace.com/2020/07/collective-trauma-amid-covid-excerpt-from-together-apart/

Kearns, M., Muldoon, O. T., Msetfi, R. M., & Surgenor, P. W. G. (2017). Darkness into Light? Identification with the Crowd at a Suicide Prevention Fundraiser Promotes Well-being Amongst Participants. *European Journal of Social Psychology, 47*(7), 878–888. https://doi.org/10.1002/ejsp.2304

Koselleck, R., & Richter, M. W. (2006). Crisis. *Journal of the History of Ideas, 67*(2), 357–400.

Lindinger-Sternart, S., Kaur, V., Widyaningsih, Y., & Patel, A. K. (2021). COVID-19 Phobia Across the World: Impact of Resilience on COVID-19 Phobia in Different Nations. *Counselling and Psychotherapy Research, 21*(2), 290–302.

Lourens, M. (2020, April 19). A Snapshot of Lockdown Shows Big Changes. *Sunday Star-Times*, 2–3.

Masten, A. S. (2001). Ordinary Magic: Resilience Processes in Development. *American Psychologist, 56*(3), 227–238.

Matthewman, S., & Huppatz, K. (2020). A Sociology of Covid-19. *Journal of Sociology, 46*(4), 675–683.

May, V. (2011). Self, Belonging and Social Change. *Sociology, 45*(3), 363–378.

Meszaros, I. (2014). *The Necessity of Social Control*. NYU Press.

Möhring, K., Naumann, E., Reifenscheid, M., Wenz, A., Rettig, T., Krieger, U., Friedel, S., Finkel, M., Cornesse, C., & Blom, A. G. (2020). The COVID-19 Pandemic and Subjective Well-being: Longitudinal Evidence on Satisfaction with Work and Family. *European Societies, 1–17*. https://doi.org/10.1080/14616696.2020.1833066

Monaghan, L. F. (2020). Coronavirus (COVID-19), Pandemic Psychology and Fractured Society: A Sociological Case of Critique Foresight and Action. *Sociology of Health & Illness, 42*(8), 1982–1995.

Monbiot, G. (2020, March 31). The Horror Films got It Wrong: This Virus has Turned us into Caring Neighbours. *The Guardian*. https://www.theguardian.com/commentisfree/2020/mar/31/virus-neighbours-covid-19

Moore, A. (2017). 'Measuring Economic Uncertainty and its Effects'. *Economic Record, 93*(303), 550–575.

Morales- Rodríguez, F. M. (2021). Fear, Stress, Resilience and Coping Strategies during COVID-19 in Spanish University Students. *Sustainability, 13*(11), 2–19.

Neal, A. G. (1998). *National Trauma and Collective Memory: Major Events in the American Century*. M. E. Sharpe, Armonk.

Nicholson, C. (2010). Children and Adolescents in Trauma. In C. Nicholson, M. Irwin, & K. N. Dwivendi (Eds.), *Creative Therapeutic Approaches*. Jessica Kingsley Publishers.

Nicola, M., Alsafi, Z., Sohrabi, C., Kerwan, A., Al-Jabir, A., Iosifidis, C., Agha, M., & Agha, R. (2020). The Socio-economic Implications of the Coronavirus Pandemic (COVID-19): A Review. *International Journal of Surgery, 78*, 185–193.

Oosterhoff, B., Palmer, C. A., Wilson, J., & Shook, N. (2020). Adolescents' Motivations to Engage in Social Distancing during the COVID-19 Pandemic: Associations with Mental and Social Health. *Journal of Adolescent Health, 67*, 179–185.

Papadopoulos, R. (2007). Refugees, Trauma and Adversity-Activated Development. *European Journal of Psychotherapy and Counselling, 9*(3), 301–312. https://doi.org/10.1080/13642530701496930

Papadopoulos, R. K. (2004). *Trauma in a Systemic Perspective: Theoretical, Organizational and Clinical Dimensions*. Paper Presented at the 14th Congress of the International Family Therapy Association, Istanbul.

Papadopoulos, R. K. (2006). Terrorism and Panic. *Psychotherapy and politics international, 4*(2), 90–100.

Pinquart, M., & Silbereisen, R. K. (2004). Human Development in Times of Social Change: Theoretical Considerations and Research Needs. *International Journal of Behavioral Development, 28*, 289–298.

Pratt, A. C. (2020). Covid-19 Impacts Cities, cultures and Societies. *City, Culture and Society., 21*, 1–2.

Ren, S. Y., Gao, R. D., & Chen, Y. L. (2020). Fear Can Be More Harmful than the Severe Acute Respiratory Syndrome Coronavirus 2 in Controlling the Coronavirus Disease 2019 Epidemic. *World Journal of Clinical Cases, 8*(4), 652–657.

Risi, E., Pronzato, R., & Fraia, G. (2020) Everything is Inside the Home: The Boundaries of Home Confinement during the Italian Lockdown. *European Societies* 1–14. https://doi.org/10.1080/14616696.2020.1828977

Rutter, M. (1994). Stress Research: Accomplishments and Tasks Ahead. In R. J. Haggerty, L. R. Sherrod, N. Garmezy, & M. Rutter (Eds.), *Stress, Risk, and Resilience in Children and Adolescents* (pp. 354–385). Cambridge University Press.

Schoon, I. (2007). Adaptations to Changing Times: Agency in Context. *International Journal of Psychology., 42*(2), 94–101.

Sennett, D. (1998). *Der flexible Mensch: Die Kultur des neuen Kapitalismus* [The Flexible Person: On the Culture of the New Capitalism] (8th ed.). Berlin: Berlin Verlag.

Silbereisen, R. K. (2005). Social Change and Human Development: Experiences from German Unification. *International Journal of Behavioral Development, 29*, 2–13.

Silbereisen, R. K., & Chen, X. (Eds.). (2010). *Social Change and Human Development: Concepts and Results*. Sage.

Silbereisen, R. K., & Eye, A. (1999). *Growing Up in Time of Social Change* (Series: International Studies on Childhood and Adolescence) (Vol. 7). De Gruyter.

Silbereisen, R. K., Pinquart, M., Reitzle, M., Tomasik, M. J., Fabel, K., & Grümer, S. (2006). Psychosocial Resources and Coping with Social Change. http://psydok.psycharchives.de/jspui/bitstream/20.500.11780/460/1/sfb_580_silbereisen_5.pdf

Spini, D., Elcheroth, G., Fasel, R., & Corkalo Biruski, D. (2014). Towards a Community Approach of the Aftermath of War in the Former Yugoslavia: Collective Experiences, Social Practices, and Representations. In D. Spini, G. Elcheroth, & D. Corkalo Biruski (Eds.), *War, Community, and Social Change: Collective Experiences in the Former Yugoslavia*. Springer.

Strong, P. (1990). Epidemic Psychology: A Model. *Sociology of Health and Illness., 12*(3), 249–259.

Tangjia, W. (2014, June). A Philosophical Analysis of the Concept of Crisis'. *Frontiers of Philosophy in China, 9*(2), 254–267.

Ungar, M. T. (2004). A Constructionist Discourse on Resilience. *Youth Society, 35*, 341–365.

United Nations (2021) Department of Economic and Social Affairs, Islam, S. N., Cheng, H. W. H., Kristinn, S, Helgason, K. S., Hunt, N., Kawamura, H., LaFleur, M., Iversen, K., & Julca, A. (2021). UN Department of Economic and Social Affairs (DESA) Working Papers (18 Jun 2021), p. 55.

Wang, C., Pan, R., Wan, X., Tan, Y., Xu, L., Ho, C. S., & Ho, R. C. (2020). Immediate Psychological Responses and Associated Factors during the Initial Stage of the 2019 Coronavirus Disease (COVID-19) Epidemic among the General Population in China. *International Journal of Environmental Research and Public Health, 17*(5), 1729.

Ward, P. R. (2020). A Sociology of the Covid-19 Pandemic: A Commentary and Research Agenda for Sociologists. *Journal of Sociology*, 1–10. https://doi.org/10.1177/1440783320939682

WHO. (2021). World Health Organisation: Social Stigma Associated with COVID-19. Retrieved June 18, 2021, from https://www.who.int/publications/m/item/a-guide-to-preventing-and-addressing-social-stigma-associated-with-covid-19?gclid=CjwKCAjwi_b3BRAGEiwAemPNUzA-jknfOIshPMXXkUYl7xkWVLxvYdtzN8mNiMqswkISReMozyhExPhoC-w3gQAvD_BwE.

Zhou, S.-J., Zhang, L.-G., Wang, L.-L., et al. (2020). Prevalence and Socio-demographic Correlates of Psychological Health Problems in Chinese Adolescents during the Outbreak of COVID-19. *European Child & Adolescent Psychiatry, 29*, 749–758.

Žižek, S. (2020). *Pandemic! Covid-19 Shakes the World*. OR Books.

3

Trauma

This chapter introduces the meaning and discusses the impact of trauma in relation to the Covid-19 pandemic by emphasising the association between trauma and loss. In order to explore this, we first provide a broad definition of trauma, followed by specific psychoanalytic explanations of the significance of loss in relation to trauma, which is rooted in childhood and especially the mother–child relationship. Specific consequences of experienced trauma are also discussed in relation to (a) symbiosis, (b) isolation and (c) disruption of time continuity. Collective trauma is also considered representing a distinct understanding of trauma.

Introduction

Trauma is a term used in everyday language to refer to individual trauma, personal trauma or collective trauma (i.e. effecting a group of people) caused by a specific harmful event. The word "trauma" comes from the Greek language, signifying a wound, an injury, a piercing of the skin or a breaking of the bodily envelope (Garland, 2002, p. 9), but Kalsched explains that "the word trauma simply refers to the fact that we are all given more to experience in this life than we can bear to experience consciously" (Kalsched, 2021, p. 444). According to Laplanche and Pontalis (1973, p. 465) in their *Dictionary of Psychoanalysis*, trauma is described as "an event in the subject's life defined by its intensity, by the subject's incapacity to respond adequately to it, and by the upheaval and long-lasting effects that it brings about in the psychical organization".[1] What is also important to characterise an event as traumatic is not only the nature of the real event, but also the psychological meaning ascribed to it.

Psychoanalytic Approaches on Trauma

The first studies on trauma come from psychoanalysis and the study of the unconscious. One of the first to define and study primarily individual trauma was Freud who defined trauma as affect that exceeds the subject's capacity for discharge (Freud, 1888/1893). Freud initially understood trauma as "a psychoenergistic imbalance caused by the breakdown of a stimulus barrier and sudden overwhelming of the psychic apparatus by powerful effects generated by an actual occurrence" (Ulman & Brothers, 1988, pp. 46–47). Later Freud considered trauma as a psychic injury in face of which the ego is overwhelmed, feeling abandoned to the situation, to excitations that are too powerful for the mental processes to deal with. So Freud, though well aware of the effects of physical trauma, moves the definition over to the mental, in other words, the piercing and wounding of the mind by events (Freud, 1916–1917). A trauma "overwhelms existing defences against anxiety in a form which provides confirmation of those deepest universal anxieties" (Garland, 2002, p. 11). Following a similar psychoanalytic approach, Caruth (1995) explained that traumatic events cannot be easily let go because they happen suddenly and rapidly and thus cannot be experienced rationally or consciously, rather they are

---

[1] Psychoanalytic Glossary (2016) offers a more clinical definition of trauma according to which, the trauma is the psychological disruption that occurs in response to a sudden overwhelming stimulus and has severe and pervasive negative impact on psychological function. The subjective mental state associated with trauma is one of helplessness, ranging from total apathy and withdrawal to emotional storm accompanied by disorganised behaviour bordering on panic. Many aspects of personality functioning may be affected including the sense of self, the quality of relations, the capacity for symbolisation and fantasy, affect tolerance, reality testing and secondary process thinking.

experienced irrationally and unconsciously and are ultimately repressed. Consequently, traumatic feelings do not derive necessarily from the harmful event *per se*, but rather from the anxiety to keep those feelings repressed. In that respect, anxiety serves as a protective mechanism against internally generated traumatic stimuli (Freud, 1926).

Freud (1926) makes a distinction between automatic and signal anxiety; automatic anxiety is a response to a real situation of danger and signal anxiety is experienced with the real threat of danger. Since a person experiences a distressing event, their capacity to distinguish between automatic and signal anxiety is suspended. Any similarity with the original event in the future may be perceived as dangerous and threatening; words, sounds, images and smells associated with the traumatising event produce overwhelming anxiety in the form of flashbacks. In the case of the pandemic, it is possible that people re-live cases of helplessness that have been experienced in a more primitive stage of life, and such re-occurrence may allow the emergence of intense emotions like the ones already identified by the relevant literature discussed previously. In fact Okorn et al. (2020) attempted to show that people who have experienced war may re-live familiar emotions (deriving from their past traumatic experiences) during the pandemic. However, we are suggesting a more general effect. This is not to say that the events of the pandemic are not provocative of anxiety or distress, but rather, that these experiences tap into and exacerbate underlying vulnerabilities which act together causing traumatic effects.

But what is the mechanism of trauma? Where does it derive from? The answer can be found within the mother–child relationship (or the child's relationship with the primary caregiver). What has widely been highlighted apart from Freud's intrapsychic conflicts is the role of external traumatic experiences. The reality of early childhood traumatic experiences and their impact on the formation of mental representations of self are emphasised by Jung, Ferenczi, Anna Freud and A. Adler. This model has been developed by followers of Freud like Klein, Winnicott, Fairbairn and Bion; they also included object relations, attachment processes and the relationships with others in the formation of the personality and pathology following trauma (Athanasiadou-Lewis, 2019).

According to psychoanalytic theories (Klein, 1932, 1952), one of the most primary traumatic experiences that may be relived through re-traumatisation is the lack of maternal care. During the first six months of life, the infant's mental capacity to experience the absence of her/his care-taker is immature. Additionally, the infant is not able yet to perceive the self and the (m)other as separate individuals; psychoanalytic theory (Klein, 1952) suggests that the infant perceives the absent mother as a bad "object" that continues to be present, but one that also attacks the baby. This is an anxiety about a fear of annihilation, experienced by the baby as a persecutory anxiety. In this position, the infant deals with this anxiety by splitting the good from the bad aspect of the object/mother and projecting the bad feelings outside of itself. The infant is intolerant towards ambivalence and so cannot integrate the bad feelings, associated with the other, with the good feelings, associated with itself. Klein calls this inner constellation the 'paranoid schizoid position'. It is a 'position' rather than only a developmental phase since it can be position taken up at later stages of life, especially in the face of conflict and stress.

This position may be relived later in life when the individual faces again a significant loss. Thus, victims of a major traumatic event may unconsciously adopt the defence of denial of their inner vulnerabilities as a means to reduce psychic pain and project them outside, to an object that is experienced as a persecuting one. Unwanted parts of oneself are projected outside, so the persecutory object resides outside of the self.

In the second half of the first year of life, the individual is gradually shifting in a position where s/he is more capable of experiencing the difference between self and other. S/he also becomes more capable of attributing good and bad aspects in the same object, which means that the mother may be good as well as bad at the same time; that opposite qualities can be seen as belonging to the same object and the object is now experienced as a whole. At this stage, aggression towards what was formerly perceived as the 'bad mother' (perceived as a quite separate object) is directed against the good mother as well, giving rise to feelings of guilt and anxiety about destroying the mother. These feelings may lead to acts of restoration against aggressive fantasies of destroying the mother. This constellation forms what Melanie Klein described as the "depressive position" (Klein, 1952). The depressive position is characterised by a greater tolerance of ambivalence and desire to make reparation for any harm. In this position, the infant encounters the reality principle—a more realistic perception of the external world, starting to perceive the object as a whole with good and bad qualities, to recognise its separate existence from one-self and to feel guilt as well that her/his destructiveness will destroy the object. While the depressive position is more associated with maturity, it is important to recognise that individuals may alternate between the paranoid-schizoid and depressive positions throughout life.

From this developmental stage emerges the capacity for sympathy and concern for others while destructive feelings are lessened. In fact, the anxieties that characterise the depressive position are a fear of destroying the other while the anxieties that characterise the previous position, the 'paranoid' one, are a fear of being destroyed. In the paranoid position, anxieties and defences are of a primitive nature while in the depressive position, defences are more mature. Immature defences include projection, splitting, projective identification, idealisation, denial and regression (Steiner, 1992, p. 47). For instance, a projection of a predominantly hostile inner world which is ruled by persecutory gears leads to the introjection of a hostile external world. *Vice versa*, the introjection of a hostile external world reinforces the projection of a hostile inner world (Klein, 1946, p. 103), and thus the manner in which the mother supports the infant to learn to moderate and manage its feelings due to a sense of safety she establishes is crucial.

Mature defences of the depressive position include intellectualisation, sublimation, humour, altruism and rationalisation. Manic defences, reparation and repression are also included in the depressive defences (Klein, 1952). Normally, individuals work through the depressive position by differentiating their aggressive fantasies from reality (i.e. differentiating aggressive thoughts from real acts of aggression). If not worked through efficiently, it may lead to excessive anxiety and guilt about the possibility of harming loved others just by having aggressive thoughts or feelings. Additionally, after successful mastering of the depressive position, the individual becomes more capable of forming interpersonal relationships, which involve the acknowledgement of aggression as an inseparable part of one's personality and by working it through.

Theorists from the object relations school such as Fairbairn, Winnicott and Balint emphasize on the interpersonal and social relationships rather than in intrapsychic conflicts. According to Fairbairn, when interpersonal or social relationships are destroyed, the child turns away from external reality and creates a fantasy of internal objects which are similar to the outside objects with which the child cannot relate in a meaningful manner (Brandell, 2012, p. 54).

Winnicott focuses on the concept of the true and false self, where the true self is the infant's core self which is developed and nourished; the false self is a façade that the child adopts to ensure compliance with the mother's inadequate responses. In Winnicott's thinking, children who are deprived from adequate care can survive but this costs them their true self; they live falsely (Young, 2004, p. 55). Balint also believes that later pathology may form on the basis of pathological responses of caregivers to the child's needs (Brandell, in Ringel and Brandell (2012), pp. 55–56). Kohut, argues that trauma is a result of chronically occurring breaches in the parental empathy, which adversely affects the relationship between child and caregiver. This can be a result of parental pathology or environmental deficits (Brandell, in Ringel & Brandell, 2012, p. 57).

As seen above, when conceptualising trauma, theorists from the object relations school emphasise interpersonal and social relationships rather than intrapsychic conflicts. Trauma links the inside with the outside, the external event with its consequences in the psychic reality. Also, in trauma, a fundamental safe and containing object relationship breaks down; in this sense, trauma is a relational concept (Bohleber, 2010, p. 98, 100). Ferenczi, one of the pioneers of the relational school maintains that one of the most traumatizing aspects of a traumatic event is its denial by the adult victimizer and especially guilt feelings that accompanies it (Ferenczi, 1980, pp. 156–167; Brandell, J. R. in Ringel & Brandell, 2012, p. 51). In this way, external reality is rejected since—according to the adult—nothing bad ever happened and the child has to rely on a distorting reality in order to survive (Athanasiadou-Lewis, C. 2019; Bohleber, 2010). These attacks on linking between reason and emotion, between inner and outer experience, are, according to Bion (1967), a key element in psychotic function. In this sense, trauma may be regarded as a relational concept, since it displays a fundamental breakdown of the relationship to a safe and containing object, leading also to a distortion between external and internal reality (Bohleber, 2010, p. 98, 100). Thus, confusing messages, acts that contradict words, words that contradict emotions, especially common among authority figures who are facing an emergency such as the pandemic (Cherry et al., 2021; Sharma, 2020; Xu and Cheng, 2021, WHO, 2022a), may trigger a distorted reality perception in some vulnerable individuals.

For example, during the first stages of the pandemic, uncertainty was mostly denied by the WHO when giving instructions of not wearing masks (Marasinghe, 2020; WHO, 2020). However, some individuals may have sensed feelings of insecurity and uncertainty among authority figures who gave such instructions, regarding their efforts to display confidence. As a result, authorities may have gotten into suspicion of hiding something. As the instructions later changed to the quite opposite (Howard et al., 2021), in a similarly confident fashion, these suspicions may have changed to paranoid beliefs that "all of this is a lie".

Another example is the so-called 'herd immunity', which would certainly prevent the virus to spread but later was found to be impractical (Brett & Rohani, 2020; WHO, 2022b; Sridhar & Gurdasani, 2021; Aschwanden, 2020). In order to achieve this, approximately 70 percent of the general population had to be immunized, preferably by vaccination (Anand & Stahel, 2021; Smith, 2019). Almost three years later, no vaccine is capable of preventing the virus to spread.

Nevertheless, the above-mentioned approaches and particularly Melanie Klein's theory may help realise the pivotal association between trauma and loss. It may also assist in distinguishing the main differences in response styles to a traumatic event which is linked to serious loss related to the pandemic. As will be further discussed, the core loss associated with the Covid-19 pandemic is the loss of lifestyle prior to the pandemic. Kalsched (2021) explains that psychological defences will be necessary to help survive traumatic experiences that people cannot yet integrate. Some individuals may react with almost complete denial of the potential loss, which may generate paranoid fears against something or someone who conspires against their integrity, which is in accordance with the paranoid-schizoid position. Others may experience intense helplessness, feelings of depression, fear or anxiety against loss or, alternatively, manic reactions of being almost invulnerable, which may be linked to difficulties in mastering the depressive position. Finally, some individuals may be capable of making more integrative experiences in terms of perceiving both bad and good aspects of an event, facing both loss and opportunities to move forward. Experiencing trauma primarily through loss may take different forms, and some of them are discussed in relation to the Covid-19 pandemic.

Consequences of Experienced Trauma

Consequences of trauma may be reflected in various aspects of peoples' lives both at conscious and unconscious levels. In this chapter, we have concentrated on three specific personal areas in which the impact of trauma may be revealed. These three areas have been chosen, following our review of the literature on the traumatic impact of Covid-19. These are 'symbiosis', 'isolation' and the 'disruption of time continuity'. The first, symbiosis, mostly mirrors intrapsychic experiences, but it is also combined with the literal meaning of symbiosis. The second, isolation, is approached as the extreme opposite of symbiosis which has frequently been revealed through studies on Covid-19. Third the disruption of time continuity, which like isolation, has also been portrayed in relation to Covid-19 through social change and crisis.

a. Symbiosis

The term symbiosis is used to refer to the feature of primitive cognitive affective life wherein the differentiation between self and (m)other has not taken place or where regression to that self-object undifferentiated state (which characterised the symbiotic phase) has recurred (Mahler et al., 1975, p. 8). Other terms used to describe undifferentiation include 'merger' (David, 1980; Jacobson, 1964; Pine, 1985), 'fusion' (Nacht, 1964; Rose, 1964, 1972), 'primary narcissism' (Grunberger, 1971), 'projective identification' (Klein, 1955) and undifferentiation itself (Stolorow & Lachman, 1980).

According to Blass and Blatt (1996), symbiosis is also an intrapsychic experience (Angel, 1967, 1972; Harrison, 1986) and can be used to define experiential states (Meissner, 1981, p. 722). The intrapsychic state of undifferentiation denoted by the concept of symbiosis can be associated with two categories of experience. (i) "The first one refers to the experience of fusion where the lack of differentiation of self and object involves the omnipotent experience of the other as part of oneself. (ii) The other category is that of merger where the lack of differentiation reflects the most intimate tie between the individual and the maternal object in which the two are experienced as joined together into one" (Blass & Blatt, 1996, p. 723).

The sense of true attachment is found in the symbiotic experience of merger which is expressed in the idea 'we are one'. In the experiences of fusion in the form of the extension of the self (Schaffer, 1968) the object is experienced as belonging to the self. "Symbiosis both as merger and as fusion may be experienced as a sense of oneness and unity because of the capacity to recognise that there is another with whom one is united" (Blass & Blatt, 1996, p. 739). Symbiosis can be divided into primary and secondary. 'Primary symbiosis' refers to the case where separation from the mother has not occurred or has taken place but only tentatively (Lewis Jr & Landis, 1973, p. 231). In secondary symbiosis, the person has achieved some degree of intrapsychic differentiation from the mother, but at the same time the person feels the need to re-establish other relationships modelled on the mother–child relationship (Lewis Jr & Landis, 1973, p. 237). This form of symbiosis characterises relationships that are pathologically intimate, resulting from the child who has never differentiated her/his own self or is unable to develop satisfactory relationships outside the family. The symbiotic person lacks of separate identity and does not experience her/himself as a differentiated self but as a part of a unity (ibid., p. 35). Symbiosis is also associated with the aspects of 'fixation' and 'regression', especially within traumatic contexts.

In cases of a traumatic incident, regression may occur and in some cases even fixation as responses to traumatic events. According to Freud (1917, p. 342), 'regression' refers to a "return from a higher to a lower stage of development". Regression occurs as a return to previous phases of development, of thought, of object relations and of behavioural structures (Laplanche & Pontalis, 1981, p. 374). Similarly, according to Meerloo (1962, p. 79), regression literally means "growing backward", to "set back the clock of development" and we also use the term to "describe the return of an organism to a less differentiated state in which it lives on a more archaic and primitive plain of behaviour" (Meerloo, 1962, p. 80). After exposure to extreme danger and stress, or shock phenomena, and especially after a trauma, states of regression may emerge and organisms tend to adopt a more primitive and less complicated form of life (ibid., p. 78). One can observe a disintegration of function and primitivisation of actions. Likewise, Meerloo (1962, p. 83) argues that "when man regressed during extreme stress, he forfeits libido and individuality and becomes a passive symbiotic animal again". An extreme of this state can be perceived through the concept of 'fixation' defined as a state of mind where the person remains absorbed in mental concentration upon the past (Freud, 1917, p. 276); it is something that resists change and does not move forward or backward.

Although the literature is limited, symbiosis can be related to the experience of Covid-19 especially during the April lockdown, as it included social isolation measures imposing people and primarily families to live under the same roof until the lifting of the measure. Some people experienced symbiosis more intensively (entail regression and fixation) whereas others experienced isolation.

b. Isolation

The Covid-19 pandemic and specifically the measures of social isolation, social distancing and the quarantine have been a traumatic experience for many, where feelings of helplessness have been generated along with fears of annihilation (Schejtman, 2021) and anxiety. Jiao et al. (2020) maintain that psychosocial distress, including depression, can result from social isolation and quarantining, arguing that social restrictions associated with Covid-19 have affected the lived experiences of the pandemic on a personal as well as a collective level. In psychoanalytic language, what contributes to the sense of loneliness is the unsatisfied longing for an understanding response without words and derives from the depressive feeling of an irretrievable loss. A satisfactory early relation with the mother is a foundation of the most complete experience of being understood (Klein, 1975). However, the happy relation with the mother is not undisturbed since destructive feelings arise in the infant and therefore the infant experiences insecurity, which is the root of loneliness. Full integration and understanding of one's emotions cannot easily be achieved and this contributes to the sense of loneliness (Klein, 1975, p. 301).

Additionally, loneliness can derive from the certainty that there is no group to which one belongs. As certain components of the self are split off, they are not available anymore and cannot be regained. These parts are projected into other people, and this contributes to the feeling that one is not in full possession of her/his own self, that one does not belong to oneself. The lost parts are felt to be lonely (Klein, 1975, p. 302). Nevertheless, being used to social isolation as a result of a way of life can make social distancing less challenging and isolation less problematic (McKenna-Plumley et al., 2021). However, isolation in particular has been more intensely experienced during the lockdown periods as it has been associated with the disruption of time, daily rhythm and continuity.

c. Disruption of Time Continuity

Nicholson (2010) argues that since human beings are programmed to function within a set of biological, rhythmic cycles, then trauma can be seen as a serious disruption of life's continuity, as a process where the repetition of everyday experiences is disrupted by a sudden event or disrupting experiences and which breaks the trust that humans have for the continuation of their life course and activities. This can lead to a lack of belief in the goodness of one's internal objects. In this sense, Schejtman (2021) claims that this pandemic has been traumatic as the continuity of everyday life has been disrupted, which in turn reactivates our feelings of helplessness, effectively increasing fears of annihilation, crises, regressions and anxiety. Those who have experienced trauma find it difficult to experience the sense of trust or objective reality and cannot trust the reliability of everyday events; they also cannot find meaning in the ordinary continuity and predictability of life. Similarly, time and the sense of time is devastated since the traumatic past seems to exist in the present (Ringel, in Ringel and Brandell, 2012, p. 74).

According to recent studies by Bonsaksen et al. (2020) and Cooke et al. (2020), the pandemic can constitute a traumatic experience leading to post-traumatic stress. The stress of the pandemic has also been found to contribute to emotional stress, sadness, fear, loneliness, anxiety and depression (Pfefferbaum & North, 2020). Such mood disorders and psychological impacts are associated with the disruption of rhythm under the stress of the pandemic (Yang et al., 2021). During the first lockdown, studies from several countries reported a feeling that time had slowed down compared to before such as France (Droit-Volet et al., 2020), Italy (Cellini et al., 2020) and the UK (Ogden, 2020). At the same time, these studies reveal that what is related to this sense of time has to do with the emotion linked to the difficulty of life during the quarantine and the disruption of life continuity due to the stop of normal life. Boredom, life rhythm and sleep quality were very much associated with the feeling that time passes slowly or stops. Due to this feeling, individuals may be prevented from planning for the future or setting goals (Lewin, 1942), which may increase the risk of depression (Abramson et al., 1989).

Social isolation measures can generate boredom, which can affect the relation individuals have with time, appearing slow, monotonous and long (Kumar & Nayar, 2020). Quarantine leads to the interruption of normal daily routine, working life and leisure activities. Losing the days and specific landmarks for each day may lead people to lose motivation (Dai & Li, 2019). At the same time, there are new activities adopted with an increase in time spent in front of a screen (Grondin et al., 2020). Research has also shown that boredom and media use were associated with an increased burden or psychological distress during Covid-19 and that the sense of meaning modified this association (Chao et al., 2020).

The way individual trauma has been depicted in literature is mainly influenced by the psychoanalytical tradition which emphasises the repressed, unconscious roots of traumatised experiences associated with loss of the fundamental connection between the infant and the mother. In this sense, Covid-19 has been approached through (limited) literature as a trigger that may allow previously suppressed traumatic experiences to re-surface especially through the experience of loss of life prior to the pandemic. Below, trauma is approached through collective experiences of adversity termed collective trauma.

Collective Trauma

Trauma that is shared by a larger group is called collective trauma in response to a mass traumatising event such as natural and other disasters or wars that impact collective identity; collective trauma refers to an entire group's psychological reaction to a traumatic event, such as the Trail of Tears (Native Americans), slavery, Japanese internment and the Holocaust. There is a psychic continuity between generations, patterns of repetition of memories transmitted intergenerationally as a form of 'haunting' (Gordon, 2008). Haunting is the power that a 'ghost' has over individuals; it can't be reduced merely to an individual's biography, loss or trauma; rather, it signifies a condition that makes biography historically possible, characterising a whole social structure and especially when losses are over (wars, etc.) (Gordon, 2008, pp. 179–184). Thus, unlike individual memory, it can persist across generations and time (Saul, 2013). Goh et al. (2020) argue that the Covid-19 pandemic has serious destructive consequential effects worldwide, particularly in deaths and economic burdens, whereas Kalsched (2021) perceives Covid-19 as an event that has caused collective as well as personal trauma as it is capable of "hijacking human imagination" through activating traumatic memories of the historical past and turn it into destructive consequences for both individuals and groups.

For Hirschberger (2018), the collective traumatic event is a cataclysmic event that shatters the basic fabric of society. In the case of the pandemic, one can speak about a 'societal trauma' which refers to a broader category of disturbance that society may experience as a result of upheavals that affects society. This implies that a whole group or society or community has been traumatised (Okorn et al., 2020). Watson et al. add that the Covid-19 pandemic is shared not only nationally but also globally as it emotionally connects people around the world through experiences of helplessness, uncertainty, loss and grief (Watson, et al., 2020). According to Nikolo (2021), collective trauma imposes itself in its raw reality and the mind cannot overcome it. In that sense, some of the features of the Covid-19 pandemic-collective trauma include its sudden character that alters our normal life and rhythms, as the patterns of lives have been disrupted causing anxiety whereas the fear of death causes a sense of precariousness (Nikolo, 2021).

Similarly, collective trauma has been depicted by Neal (1998) as the collective response to a traumatising event (an earthquake, volcano eruption etc.) which causes radical change and disruption within a short period of time although Erikson (1976) maintains that collective trauma refers to a shock of gradual change of social life that damages the bond that allows people to form relations; it is thus understood through the lived experiences of people who survived it and does not entail the element of sudden change like individual trauma.

Kalsched (2021) depicts the Covid-19 pandemic as a collective traumatic experience as it involves the experience of collective traumas like the isolation and loneliness during periods of quarantine, the fear of death, the loss of a dependable future and economic anxieties. Brooks et al. (2020) add that changes imposed because of the Covid-19 pandemic, such as lockdown, social distancing, stay-at-home policies, travel restrictions, social isolation and quarantines, were adopted leading to increased vulnerabilities regarding mental health associated with posttraumatic symptoms. Okorn et al. (2020) maintain that such collective traumas may 'trigger' some people's un-remembered, suppressed past injuries and experiences like war.

Nevertheless, events may be traumatic themselves, however, "mere existence of certain devastating events should not lead to a conclusion that every person exposed to them is likely to be psychologically traumatized" (Papadopoulos, 2007, p. 304) as different people experience external devastating events in very different ways that depend on many different factors. Most individuals do not require specialist attention after experiencing a traumatic event as their functioning remains intact and unaffected; therefore it does not change either positively or negatively. Alexander (2012) explains that although trauma is mainly perceived as emerging from events themselves, events characterised as traumatic do not necessarily create collective trauma as trauma is a socially mediated attribution which can be ascribed as such before or after the harmful event. Thus for Papadopoulos (2007), different people react differently to the same traumatic event, whereas for Alexander (2012), collective trauma does not necessarily derive from every traumatic event. Collective trauma for Alexander is not the result of a group experiencing pain; processes of social change, even while causing social disruption, do not necessarily cause collective social traumas.

In order for collective trauma to emerge, social crises must become cultural crises. For Alexander, cultural trauma can be depicted as a discomfort entering into a collective meaning-making of identity. Group members represent social pain as a fundamental component of who they are (e.g. Holocaust). Cultural construction of trauma is thus formed through a narrative about a "horribly destructive social process and a demand for emotional, institutional and symbolic separation and reconstruction" (Alexander, 2012, p. 16). Along the same lines, Demertzis and Eyerman (2020) referred to cultural trauma which "occurs as the taken for granted foundations of individuals and collective identity are shattered, setting in motion a discursive process to understand what happened, assign blame and find pathways to repair an interpreted situation". Cultural trauma is a specific form of collective trauma affecting collective identity where groups of individuals feel similarly affected by the fracture of the existential security that a sense of identity offers. Similarly, Baquero (2021, p. 6) maintains that trauma is "extended to a social group depending on how it has been socially depicted through narratives and media. It is a result of social and cultural narration of social suffering which requires understanding, interpretation and representation". In the case of the Covid-19 pandemic, it seems hard to refer to a 'cultural trauma' due to its global magnitude. Lack of relevant literature limits the attempt of the current section to portray the traumatic components of the Covid-19 pandemic. However, taking Papadopoulos and Alexander into account, we should be very careful in classifying Covid-19 as a 'collective' or more specifically 'cultural' trauma although traumatic events have certainly been associated with this pandemic through its analysis as radical change and global crisis affecting and transforming people, lives and societies.

Although (limited) relevant literature has identified the Covid-19 pandemic as a collective trauma associated with shared traumatic experiences, this section also discussed approaches that may prevent us from such a generalisation. What remains evident, however, is that the pandemic has been depicted in terms of social change and crisis entailing traumatic elements in terms of harmful events, traumatic consequences especially in relation to collective loss of life prior to the pandemic.

Synopsis

This chapter attempted a theoretical overview of the meaning and consequences of trauma within the Covid-19 context. Although literature on trauma during the pandemic has been limited, this chapter offered a comprehensive theorisation of trauma by employing psychoanalytic perspectives. It became understood that trauma is associated with prior life experiences rooted in childhood and particularly the mother-child relationship. However, we need to keep in mind that it is not necessary for an external event deriving from early life to cause a trauma; rather the importance lies with how this is understood and responded to. Even the Kleinian approach is a 'meaning-making' one, which can become a template for meaning-making in later life. Within this frame, trauma has been depicted as the meaning ascribed to the loss of the relationship between the mother and the child, or in other words, the loss of a previous, protected stage of life. Consequences of trauma have been discussed with reference to (a) symbiosis, (b) isolation and (c) disruption of time continuity. Finally, collective trauma has been depicted in terms of shared experienced trauma, although it became understood that different perspectives offer different definitions of the significance and relevance of this term, especially in relation to its contextual emergence. Still, trauma has been depicted primarily through the essence of loss and regarding the Covid-19 context it has been primarily associated with the loss of life one knew prior to the pandemic.

The following chapter will present the methodological approaches followed in this study and more importantly, will introduce the unique sample of participants involved, by offering a broad view on why, how, where and when participants' lived experiences of the Covid-19 pandemic have been researched.

Bibliography

Abramson, L. Y., Metalsky, G. I., & Alloy, L. B. (1989). Hopelessness Depression: A Theory-Based Subtype of Depression. *Psychological Review, 96*, 358–372. https://doi.org/10.1037/0033-295X.96.2.358

Alexander, J. (2012). *Trauma: A Social Theory*. Polity.

Anand, P., & Stahel, V. P. (2021). Review the Safety of Covid-19 mRNA Vaccines: A Review. *Patient Saf Surg. 1*, 15(1), 20. https://doi.org/10.1186/s13037-021-00291-9. Erratum in: *Patient Saf Surg.* 2021 May 18, 15(1), 22. PMID: 33933145; PMCID: PMC8087878.

Angel, K. (1967). On Symbiosis and Pseudosymbiosis. *Journal of American Psychoanalytic Association, 15*, 294–315.

Angel, K. (1972). The Role of the Internal Object and External Object in Object-relationships, Separation Anxiety, Object Constancy and Symbiosis. *International Journal of Psychoanalysis, 53*, 541–546.

Aschwanden, C. (2020). The False Promise of Herd Immunity. Retrieved June 20, 2022, from https://www.nature.com/articles/d41586-020-02948-4

Athanasiadou-Lewis, C. (2019). A Relational Perspective on Psychological Trauma: The Ghost of the Unspent Love. In A. Starcevic (Ed.), *Psychological Trauma*. IntechOpen. https://doi.org/10.5772/intechopen.77651

Baquero, R. P. (2021). From Psychoanalysis to Cultural Trauma: Narrating Legacies of Collective Suffering. *Critical Horizons*. https://doi.org/10.1080/14409917.2021.1957359

Bion, W. R. (1967). Attacks on Linking. In *Second Thoughts* (pp. 93–109). Jason Aronson.

Blass, R. B., & Blatt, S. J. (1996). Attachment and Separateness in the Experience of Symbiotic Relatedness. *The Psychoanalytic Quarterly, 65*(4), 711–746. https://doi.org/10.1080/21674086.1996.11927513

Bohleber, W. (2010). Destructiveness, Intersubjectivity and Trauma. In *The Identity Crisis of Modern Psychoanalysis* (pp. 75–100). Karnac Books.

Bonsaksen, T., Heir, T., Schou-Bredal, I., Ekeberg, Ø., Skogstad, L., & Grimholt, T. K. (2020). Post-traumatic Stress Disorder and Associated Factors During the Early Stage of the COVID-19 Pandemic in Norway. *International Journal of Environmental Research and Public Health, 17*, 9210. https://doi.org/10.3390/ijerph17249210

Brandell, J. R. (2012). Psychoanalytic Theory (Part I). In S. Ringel & J. R. Brandell (Eds.), *Trauma: Contemporary Directions in Theory, Practice, and Research* (pp. 41–62). Sage Publications.

Brett, T. S., & Rohani, P. (2020). Transmission Dynamics Reveal the Impracticality of COVID-19 Herd Immunity Strategies. *PNAS, 117*(41), 25897–25903. https://doi.org/10.1073/pnas.2008087117

Brooks, S. K., Webster, R. K., Smith, L. E., Woodland, L., Wessely, S., Greenberg, N., & Rubin, G. J. (2020). The Psychological Impact of Quarantine and How to Reduce It: Rapid Review of the Evidence. *Lancet, 395,* 912–920.

Caruth, C. (1995). Unclaimed Experience: Trauma Narrative and History. In C. Caruth (Ed.), *Trauma: Explorations in Memory.* John Hopkins University Press.

Cellini, N., Canale, N., Mioni, G., & Costa, S. (2020). Changes in Sleep Pattern, Sense of Time and Digital Media Use During COVID-19 Lockdown in Italy. *Journal of Sleep Research, 29,* e13074. https://doi.org/10.1111/jsr.13074

Chao, M., Chen, X., Liu, T., Yang, H., & Hall, B. J. (2020). Psychological Distress and State Boredom During the Covid-19 Outbreak in China: The Role of Meaning in Life and Media Use. *European Journal of Psychotraumatology, 11*(1), 1769379.

Cherry, T. L., James, A. G., & Murphy, J. (2021). The Impact of Public Health Messaging and Personal Experience on the Acceptance of Mask Wearing During the COVID-19 Pandemic. *Journal of Economic Behavior and Organisation, 187,* 415–430.

Cooke, J. E., Eirich, R., Racine, N., & Madigan, S. (2020). Prevalence of Posttraumatic and General Psychological Stress During COVID-19: A Rapid Review and Meta-analysis. *Psychiatry Research, 292,* 113347. https://doi.org/10.1016/j.psychres.2020.113347

Dai, H., & Li, C. (2019). How Experiencing and Anticipating Temporal Landmarks Influence Motivation. *Current Opinion in Psychology., 26,* 44–48. https://doi.org/10.1016/j.copsyc.2018.04.012

David, C. (1980). Metapsychological Reflections on the Stage of Being in Love. In S. Lebovici & D. Widlocher (Eds.), *Psychoanalysis in France* (pp. 87–109). International Universities Press.

Demertzis, N., & Eyerman, R. (2020). Covid-19 As Cultural Trauma. *American Journal of Cultural Sociology, 8,* 428–450. https://doi.org/10.1057/s41290-020-00112-z

Droit-Volet, S., Gil, S., Martinelli, N., Andant, N., Clinchamps, M., Parreira, L., et al. (2020). Time and Covid-19 Stress in the Lockdown Situation: Time Free, «Dying» of Boredom and Sadness. *PLoS One, 15,* e0236465. https://doi.org/10.1371/journal.pone.0236465

Erikson, K. (1976). *Everything in its Path: Destruction on Community in the Buffalo Creek Flood*. Simon and Schuster.

Ferenczi, S. (1980). The Confusion of Tongues between Adults and the Child: The Language of Tenderness and Passion. In M. Balint, E. Mosbacher, et al. (Eds.), *Final Contributions to the Problems and Methods of Psycho-Analysis* (pp. 156–167). Karnac Books.

Freud, S. (1893). Charcot. *The Standard Edition of the Complete Psychological Works of Sigmund Freud, 3*, 7–23.

Freud, S. (1917). Introductory Lectures on Psycho-Analysis. In *The Standard Edition of the Complete Psychological Works of Sigmund Freud*, Volume XVI (1916–1917): Introductory Lectures on Psycho-Analysis (Part III), 241–463.

Freud, S. (1926). Inhibitions, Symptoms and Anxiety. *The Standard Edition of the Complete Psychological Works of Sigmund Freud, 20*, 75–176.

Garland, C. (2002). *Understanding Trauma: A Psychoanalytical Approach*. Karnac Books. Second Enlarged Edition. First published in 1998

Goh, K. K., Lu, M. L., & Jou, S. (2020). 'Impact of COVID-19 Pandemic: Social Distancing and the Vulnerability to Domestic Violence. *Psychiatry and Clinical Neurosciences, 74*(11), 612–613.

Gordon, A. (2008). *Ghostly Matters Haunting and the Sociological Imagination*. University of Minnesota Press.

Grondin, S., Mendoza-Duran, E., & Rioux, P. A. (2020). Pandemic, Quarantine, and Psychological Time. *Frontiers in Psychology, 11*, 581036. https://doi.org/10.3389/fpsyg.2020.581036

Grunberger, B. (1971). *Narcissism: Psychoanalytic Essays*. International Universities Press.

Harrison, I. B. (1986). On "merging" and the Phantasy of Merging. *Psychoanalytic Study of the Child, 41*, 155–170.

Hirschberger, G. (2018). Collective Trauma and the Social Construction of Meaning. *Frontiers in Psychology, 9*, 1–14.

Howard, J., Huang, A., Zhiyuan Li, A. H., Tufekci, Z., Zdimal, V., van der Westhuizen, H.-M., von Delft, A., Price, A., Fridman, L., Tang, L.-H., Tang, V., Watson, G. L., Bax, C. E., Shaikh, R., Questier, F., Hernandez, D., Chu, L. F., Ramirez, C. M., Rimoin, A., et al. (2021). An Evidence Review of Face Masks Against COVID-19. *PNAS, 118*(4), e2014564118.

Jacobson, E. (1964). *The Self and the Object World*. International Universities Press.

Jiao, W. Y., Wang, L. N., Liu, J., Fang, S. F., Jiao, F. Y., Pettoello-Mantovani, M., & Somekh, E. (2020). Behavioral and Emotional Disorders in Children during the COVID-19 Epidemic. *The Journal of Pediatrics, 17*(3), 230–233.

Kalsched, D. (2021). Intersections of Personal vs. Collective Trauma during the COVID-19 Pandemic: The Hijacking of the Human Imagination. *Journal of Analytical Psychology, 66*(3), 443–462.

Klein, M. (1932). The Significance of Early Anxiety-Situations in the Development of the Ego. *The Psycho-Analysis of Children, 22*, 245–267.

Klein, M. (1946). Notes on Some Schizoid Mechanisms. *International Journal of Psychoanalysis, 27*, 99–110.

Klein, M. (1952). The Origins of Transference. *International Journal of Psychoanalysis, 33*, 433–438.

Klein, M. (1955). On Identification. In *Envy and Gratitude: A Study of Unconscious Sources* (pp. 141–175). Delacorte Press.

Klein, M. (1975). Envy and Gratitude and Other Works 1946–1963: Edited By: M. Masud R. Khan. *The International Psycho-Analytical Library* 104:1–346.

Kumar, A., & Nayar, K. R. (2020). COVID 19 and Its Mental Health Consequences. *Journal of Mental Health, 27*, 1–2. https://doi.org/10.1080/09638237.2020.1757052

Laplanche, J., & Pontalis, J. B. (1973). The Language of Psycho-Analysis: Translated by Donald Nicholson-Smith. *The Language of Psycho-Analysis, 94*, 1–497.

Laplanche, J., & Pontalis, J. B. (1981). *Leksilogio tis psichanalisis [The Dictionary of Psychoanalysis]*. Kedros Publications.

Lewin, K. (1942). Time Perspective and Morale. In G. Watson (Ed.), *Civilian Morale* (pp. 48–70). Houghton Mifflin.

Lewis, A. B., Jr., & Landis, B. (1973). Symbiotic Pairings in Adults. *Contemporary Psychoanalysis, 9*(2), 230–249. https://doi.org/10.1080/00107530.1973.10745277

Mahler, M. S., Pine, F., & Bergman, A. (1975). *The Psychological Birth of the Human Infant: Symbiosis and Individuation*. Basic Books.

Marasinghe, K. M. (2020). Face Mask Use Among Individuals Who Are Not Medically Diagnosed with COVID-19: A Lack of Evidence for and Against and Implications around Early Public Health Recommendations. *International Journal of One Health, 6*(2), 109–117. https://doi.org/10.14202/IJOH.2020.109-117

McKenna-Plumley, P. E., Graham-Wisener, L., Berry, E., & Groarke, J. M. (2021). Connection, Constraint, and Coping: A Qualitative Study of Experiences of Loneliness During the COVID-19 Lockdown in the UK. *PLoS ONE, 16*(10), e0258344. https://doi.org/10.1371/journal.pone.0258344

Meerloo, J. (1962). The Dual Meaning of Human Regression. *Psychoanalytic Review, 49*(3), 77–86.

Meissner, W. W. (1981). Metapsychology—Who Needs It? *Journal of American Psychoanalytic Association, 29,* 921–938.

Nacht, S. (1964). Silence as an Integrative Factor. *International Journal of Psychoanalysis., 45,* 299–303.

Neal, A. G. (1998). *National Trauma and Collective Memory: Major Events in the American Century.* M. E. Sharpe, Armonk.

Nicholson, C. (2010). *Children and Adolescents in Trauma. Creative Therapeutic Approaches* (C. Nicholson, M. Irwin, & K. N. Dwivendi, Eds.). Jessica Kingsley Publishers.

Nikolo, A. M. (2021). The COVID 19 Pandemic and Individual and Collective Trauma. *International Journal of Applied Psychoanalytic Studies, 1,* 1–6.

Ogden, R. S. (2020). The Passage of Time During the UK Covid-19 Lockdown. *PLoS One, 15,* e0235871. https://doi.org/10.1371/journal.pone.0235871

Okorn, I., Jahović, S., Dobranić-Posavec, M., Mladenović, J., & Glasnović, A. (2020). Isolation in the COVID-19 Pandemic as Re-traumatization of War Experiences. *Croatian Medical Journal, 61,* 371–376.

Papadopoulos, R. (2007). Refugees, Trauma and Adversity-Activated Development. *European Journal of Psychotherapy and Counselling, 9*(3), 301–312. https://doi.org/10.1080/13642530701496930

PEP Consolidated Psychoanalytic Glossary. (2016). Produced by: Psychoanalytic Electronic Publishing. https://pep-web.org/browse/document/zbk.069.0000a

Pfefferbaum, B., & North, C. S. (2020). Mental Health and the Covid-19 Pandemic. *The New England Journal of Medicine, 383*(6), 510–512. https://doi.org/10.1056/NEJMp2008017

Pine, F. (1985). *Developmental Theory and Clinical Process.* Yale University Press.

Ringel, S. (2012). Psychoanalytic Theory (Part II). In S. Ringel & J. R. Brandell (Eds.), *Trauma. Contemporary Directions in Theory, Practice, and Research* (pp. 62–77). Sage Publications.

Rose, G. J. (1964). Creative Imagination in Terms of ego 'core' and Boundaries. *International Journal of Psychoanalysis., 45,* 75–84.

Rose, G. J. (1972). Fusion States. In P. L. Giovaccini (Ed.), *Tactics and Techniques in Psychoanalytic Psychotherapy* (pp. 170–188). Science House.

Saul, J. (2013). *Collective Trauma, Collective Healing: Promoting Community Resilience in the Aftermath of Disaster* (Vol. 48). Routledge.

Schaffer, R. (1968). *Aspects of Internalization*. International Universities Press.

Schejtman, C. R. (2021). Coping with Pandemic, Psychoanalytical Interventions with Parents and Children: Institutional and Community Approaches. *International Journal of Applied Psychoanalytic Studies, 18*(2), 177–187.

Sharma, S. K. (2020). Who Should Use a Face Mask During COVID-19 Pandemic? An Evidence-based Review. *Indian Source of Respiratory Care, 9*(2), 149–152.

Smith, D. (2019, November). Herd Immunity in Veterinary Clinics of North America: Food Animal Practice in the Veterinary Clinics of North America. *Food Animal Practice, 35*(3), 593–604.

Sridhar D., & Gurdasani, D. (2021). Herd Immunity by Infection is Not An Option. Retrieved June 20, 2022, from https://www.science.org/doi/10.1126/science.abf7921

Steiner, J. (1992). The Equilibrium Between the Paranoid-Schizoid and the Depressive Positions. *Clinical Lectures on Klein and Bion, 14*, 46–58.

Stolorow, R. D., & Lachman, F. M. (1980). *Psychoanalysis and Developmental Arrest: Theory and Treatment*. International Universities Press.

Ulman, R. B., & Brothers, D. (1988). *The Shattered Self—A Psychoanalytic Study of Trauma*. The Analytic Press.

Watson, M. F., Bacigalupe, G., Daneshpour, M., Han, W. J., & Parra-Cardona, R. (2020). COVID-19 Interconnectedness: Health Inequity, the Climate Crisis, and Collective Trauma. *Family Process., 59*(2), 832–843.

WHO. (2022a). Retrieved June 20, 2022, from https://www.voanews.com/a/science-health_coronavirus-outbreak_who-dont-wear-face-masks/6186669.html

WHO. (2022b). Retrieved June 20, 2022, from https://www.who.int/news-room/questions-and-answers/item/herd-immunity-lockdowns-and-covid-19

Xu, P., & Cheng, J. (2021). Individual Differences in Social Distancing and Mask-wearing in the Pandemic of COVID-19: The Role of Need for Cognition, Self-control and Risk Attitude. *Personality and Individual Differences, 175*, 110706.

Yang, M., He, P., Xu, X., Li, D., Wang, J., Wang, Y., Wang, B., Wang, W., Zhao, M., Lin, H., Deng, M., Deng, T., Kuang, L., & Chen, D. (2021). Disrupted Rhythms of Life, Work and Entertainment and Their Associations with Psychological Impacts Under the Stress of the COVID-19 Pandemic: A Survey in 5854 Chinese People with different Sociodemographic Backgrounds. *PloS one, 16*(5), e0250770. https://doi.org/10.1371/journal.pone.0250770

Young, M. (2004). *Exploring the Meaning of Trauma in the South African Police Service.* Submitted in partial fulfilment of the requirements for the degree PhD (Psychotherapy) in the Department of Psychology at the University of Pretoria, pp. 32–56.

4

Methodological and Methodical Processes

So far, we have tried to conceptualise the meaning of change, crisis and trauma by concentrating on sociological as well as psychosocial approaches. At the same time we have attempted to contextualise these concepts within the frame of the Covid-19 pandemic. The next step is to portray the methodological approach followed in this study, the methods employed in order to collect and analyse data, and introduce the participants in terms of their sociodemographic characteristics.

Methodological Considerations

This study has been conducted by two Greek female researchers affiliated to related albeit distinct disciplines. One is trained to conduct empirical research through sociological perspectives, whereas the other is trained to employ psychosocial and more specifically psychoanalytic approaches. This combination offered a fruitful synergy of two different approaches, as the first researcher has been more concentrated on the impact of social circumstances upon lived experiences, whereas the second has been focused on the ways individuals may process and integrate such lived experiences. By combining these viewpoints, this study ultimately aims at contributing to a rounded understanding of the meaning-making of Covid-19 through lived experience of the April 2020 lockdowns. In order for this endeavour to be accomplished, we needed to employ the most enabling epistemological approach.

Interpretive phenomenology presents a unique methodology for studying lived experience as it brings to light what is often taken for granted while allowing the emergence of phenomena from the perspective of how people interpret and attribute meaning to their existence; phenomenology and more specifically hermeneutics focus on the interpretation of meaning through lived experience (Polit & Beck, 2012). The study of lived experience allows and enables the experienced aspect to make a special impression that gives it lasting importance. Lived experiences are deemed incomplete while remaining descriptive; interpretation of significance for the person and contextualisation of the social circumstances is pivotal (Gadamer, 1976, 2004). A person's life story has two dimensions that contribute to its forward movement or directedness: a chronological sequence of episodes and a construction of "meaningful totalities out of scattered events" (Ricoeur, 1981, p. 240). As this study aims at exploring the meaning-making of Covid-19 lived experiences, interpretive phenomenology offers the ideal epistemological foundations in order to describe, understand and explain the meaning-making of the pandemic through the ways participants have experienced the April 2020 lockdowns in different parts of the world.

This study is exploratory and interpretative in nature, and the purpose was not to ensure a representative or random sample; rather qualitative approach was employed in order to produce a valuable amount of rich first-hand data and to facilitate theory generation. It would therefore be more appropriate to refer to this study as an exploratory investigation (Hoaglin et al., 1983) which reveals possible tendencies concerning the meaning-making Greek people ascribed to Covid-19 through their lived experiences of the pandemic. The use of in-depth semi-structured interviews is a well-established approach to grasp the perspectives of individuals, thereby capturing their thoughts, feelings, expectations and behaviours (Esterberg, 2002) and thus exploring the inner world (in terms of meanings, feelings, beliefs) as well as the experienced social reality of the participants (Alvesson, 2002).

Methods of Data Collection

The study followed the ethical standards stipulated by the British Sociological Association guidelines on ethical research (BSA, 2022) concerning consent, anonymity, respect for participants, integrity and safe data storage. The research questions addressed during interviews were informed by the research literature and were asked in an open-ended format (Light et al., 1990; Kvale, 1996), concerned solely with personal experiences of everyday living (Baker, 1997; Roseneil & Budgeon. 2004). The questions were phrased in neutral ways asking participants to describe their everyday routines during the lockdown, deliberately avoiding any reference to the core concepts of crisis and trauma (thus limiting bias) and keeping for last the question 'what does this pandemic mean to you?'. This last question proved to be remarkably revealing, as participants had the chance to reflect upon their earlier responses and become even more detailed and thorough. Each interview lasted between 30 and 60 minutes, was conducted in Greek and/or English and coded to identify themes related to the aims of the study, through open coding techniques; contiguity-based relations between themes were identified revealing relations among parts of transcribed texts (Maxwell, 2013).

Data has been collected and transcribed by the two authors who have continually checked and reviewed the themes emerging from the data throughout the process. This approach was deemed effective to explore novel phenomena within a continuous interaction between theory generation and empirical observation (Charmaz & Belgrave, 2015). Additionally, both researchers were themselves experiencing a strict lockdown in the city of Athens, Greece, during data collection. Conscious efforts were made to remain as open and accepting as possible to different experiences participants shared while respecting and empathising with the difficulties and challenges they have been sharing, as many of the experiences were also identified in the lives of the researchers. These circumstances required the researchers to become self-reflexive and self-conscious of their own emotional and mental state during the period of data collection.

Participants: Who Are They?

To explore the meaning-making of the Covid-19 pandemic, 46 semi-structured, in-depth interviews (Maxwell, 2013) were conducted online (through Skype, messenger and WhatsApp conference platforms), during lockdowns of April 2020, given the inability to conduct the interviews face to face due to distancing measures (Jowett, 2021). The sample consisted of Greek men and women (born and raised in Greece), 24 of them residing in 6 different Greek cities and 22 of them residing in 17 cities abroad (as first-generation immigrants), including the following countries: Iceland, the UK, Belgium, Austria, Denmark, Germany, France, the Netherlands, the USA, Japan, Hong Kong and Bahrein.

The reason this sample consisted of Greek nationals living within and outside Greece relates with our attempt to explore whether the meaning-making of this pandemic might be collective among people who share common cultural experiences instead of regional similarities. We selected Greek participants as both authors are Greeks, albeit living abroad, thus we utilised the advantage of our own socio-cultural background, nationality and consequent networking. This study perceived those participants living in places other than Greece as a sort of 'control group' which enabled us to consider whether they experience lockdowns similarly to the country they are in, or alongside their Greek peers.

Participants, were aged between 21 and 84 years old, were selected based on their willingness to participate in the study, as this is commonly deemed suitable with exploratory and non-probabilistic research designs (Ritchie et al., 2013) (see Table 4.1). The sample was opportunistic as the recruitment strategy used "gatekeepers" and "snowballing" techniques (Becker, 1963), with some of the participants introducing the researcher to others.

Table 4.1 Sociodemographic data (Greece: 24 (6 cities); Diaspora: 22 (17 cities))

Name/participant	Gender	Residence	Age	Educational status	Family status	Employment status
1. Giannis	M	Japan, Tokyo	59	BA	Married 1 child	Employed, FT Director
2. Aggeliki	F	Greece, Athens	46	Postgraduate	In relationship, expecting	Employed, FT Admin
3. Michalis	M	Greece, Athens	48	Secondary	In relationship, expecting	Self-employed
4. Antigoni	F	Greece, Athens	60	Secondary	Single	Suspended
5. Nikos	M	Greece, Athens	70	Secondary	Married	Retired
6. Aristea	F	Greece, Athens	65	Secondary	Married	Housewife
7. Betty	F	Greece, Athens	75	University	Window	Retired
8. Maria	F	Greece, Athens	68	Secondary	Married/2 children	Retired
9. Mary	F	Greece, Heraklion	66	Secondary	Married/2 children	Retired
10. Dinos	M	Greece, Athens	84	Secondary	Married/1 child	Retired
11. Natalia	F	UK, Northampton	29	College	In relationship	Suspended
12. Theo	M	UK, Northampton	40	College student	In relationship	Student
13. Alina	F	UK, London	39	PhD	Married	Employed
14. Eleni	F	Japan, Tokyo	29	MSc	Married	Suspended
15. Alex	M	Denmark, Copenhagen	28	MSc	Single	Employed
16. Iason	M	Denmark, Copenhagen	28	BSc	Single	Unemployed
17. Argiro	F	Reykjavik/Iceland	40	BA	Married	Employed/subsidised
18. Marina	F	UK/London	40	MSc	Married/2 kids	Employed
19. Lia	F	Belgium, Brussels	28	BA	Single	Employed

(continued)

Table 4.1 (continued)

Name/participant	Gender	Residence	Age	Educational status	Family status	Employment status
20. Nikos	M	Eindhoven, Netherlands	26	BSc	Single	Employed
21. Sotiria	F	Reykjavik, Iceland	31	MSc	Single	Employed/subsidised
22. Koralia	F	Bahrein	40	MSc	Married/3 kids	Unemployed/housewife
23. Aggelos	M	USA, Los Angeles	24	MSc	Single	PT employed
24. Paris	M	Japan, Yokohama	36	MSc	Single	Student
25. Bill	M	USA, Maryland	78	Secondary	Married	Retired
26. Mari	F	Hong Kong	40	University	Married/1 kid	Unemployed/housewife
27. Nora	F	Greece, Athens	42	MSc	Single	Employed (public sector)
28. Aris	M	Greece, Athens	42	PhD	Married, 1 kid	Employed
29. Achilleas	M	Greece, Athens	58	Technical school	Single	Unemployed
30. Evi	F	Greece, Athens	21	University student	In relationship	Student
31. Panos	M	Greece, Athens	21	University student	In relationship	Student
32. Thanos	M	Greece, Kastoria	36	PhD	Single	Employed (NGO)
33. Ksenia	F	Greece, Athens	23	Private school	Single	Suspended
34. Kiki	F	Greece, Athens	31	MSc	Single	Employed (NGO)
35. Nikolas	M	Greece, Rhodes	35	BSc	Single	Suspended
36. Kelly	F	Greece, Athens	43	IEK	Divorced, 2 kids	Unemployed
37. Voula	F	Austria, Gratz	42	MSc	Married, 1 kid	Suspended
38. Kostas	M	Greece, Athens	60	High school	Divorced, 2 kids	Employed
39. Elena	F	Greece, Athens	35	PhD	Single, expecting	Employed, freelancer

40. Rita	F	Germany, Munich	35	Medical school	Single	Employed, doctor
41. Thalia	F	Belgium, Brussels	26	Uni student	Single	Student
42. Angela	F	Greece, Corfu	37	BSc	Divorced	Suspended
43. Zenia	F	Greece, Chania	38	Polytechnic Uni	Single	Employed, freelancer
44. Kyriakos	M	France, Paris	36	BSc	Single	Employed (NGO)
45. Andreas	M	Belgium, Brussels	27	MSc student	Single	Master student
46. Alice	F	Greece, Athens	47	MSc	Married	Medical doctor

[a]Suspended: during the pandemic, employers had the option to suspend employees, meaning that they would stop working and would receive a supplementary allowance by the government. This measure was employed in many countries. At the time data was collected, the participants who were suspended did not know if they would be offered their jobs back or not

The three tables present the collected data in two different ways. The first one includes all participants and provides a brief sociodemographic overview of each one of them, including gender, location of residence, age, educational background, family status and employment status. These characteristics were also integrated in the analysis chapters, in order to identify possible patterns associated with sociodemographic characteristics wherever relevant. Such patterns were identified in relation to specific thematic categories, found in each chapter respectively.

Tables 4.2 and 4.3 present participants residing within and outside Greece separately, allowing a comparative overview of the data. As can be seen, the demographics of the participants may differ as the 'Greek' sample is more diverse, especially in terms of age range, whereas the 'Diaspora' sample is more diverse in terms of location of residence. Only limited patterns associated with location of residence have been identified in the two analysis chapters. This observation possibly implies that shared experiences between participants have not been limited to regional specifications.

Table 4.2 Greeks living in Greece (total: 24)

(a) **Age** (21–84)
(b) **Family status** (married = 7, single = 11, in relationship = 6, window = 1, divorced = 3, parents = 6, expecting = 3)
(c) **Gender** (females = 15, males = 9)
(d) **Employment status** (employed/subsidised = 10, part time = 0, suspended = 4, unemployed = 2 housewives = 1, students = 2, retired = 5)
(e) **Educational status** (secondary education = 9, college/technical education = 3, university = 6, postgraduate = 3, PhD = 3)
(f) **Locations within Greece:** Athens = 19, Heraklion = 1, Chania = 1, Rhodes = 1, Kastoria = 1, Corfu = 1

Table 4.3 Greek Diaspora (total: 22)

(a) **Age** (24–78)
(b) **Family status** (married = 9, Single = 11, in relationship = 6, window = 0, divorced = 0, parents = 5, expecting = 0)
(c) **Gender** (females = 12, males = 10)
(d) **Employment status** (employed/subsidised = 10, part time = 1, suspended = 3, unemployed = 1, housewives = 2, students = 4, retired = 1)
(e) **Educational status** (secondary education = 1, college/technical education = 2, university = 8, postgraduate = 10, PhD = 1)
(f) **Locations abroad:** Japan/Tokyo = 2, Japan/Yokohama/1, UK/London = 2, UK/Northampton = 2, Denmark/Copenhagen = 2, Iceland/Reykjavik = 2, Belgium/Brussels = 3, Netherlands/Eindhoven = 1, Bahrein = 1, USA/LA = 1, USA/Maryland = 1, Hong Kong = 1, Austria/Gratz = 1, Germany/Munich = 1, France/Paris = 1

Analysis

Interpretative phenomenology allows the employment of different data analysis techniques. Following a hermeneutical approach, specific questions have been used during data analysis in order to enable a dialogue with the text (Gadamer, 1981). Such questions aim at identifying the ways that the phenomenon (the meaning-making about Covid-19) is being expressed in a specific encounter (though lived experiences), as well as the meaning for the interviewee and the researcher (of the lived experiences) in relation to the studied phenomenon (meaning-making of Covid-19). The process requires continued reflexive awareness of the new understanding that emerges while these questions are answered, and since this process allows themes to emerge then a thematic analysis of the data becomes particularly relevant and advantageous.

Thematic analysis (Ryan & Bernard, 2003) consisted of repeated readings of the (translated) transcripts of the interviews, focusing on meaningful and relevant categories and themes associated with lived experiences of social change, crisis and trauma during the pandemic lockdown. Contiguity-based relations between themes were identified revealing relations among parts of transcribed texts (Maxwell, 2013). The identification of these themes (formed after the completion of the initial transcript analysis) allowed the emergence of the actual connection between the concepts of social change, crisis and trauma with the Covid-19 pandemic context. Themes emerged as a part of participants' responses to the questions regarding their views on the way they lived their lives during the first pandemic lockdown.

Notably, Chap. 6 followed a supplementary analytical approach deriving from psychoanalytic theory; Frosh and Saville Young (2011) and Frosh (2010), as psychosocial thinkers, suggest a multi-level approach to data analysis including identifying core narratives in the interviews (Frosh & Emerson, 2004; Hollway & Jefferson, 2000) in different levels. As trauma has been perceived in Chap. 6 primarily through loss of the ways people lived their life prior to the pandemic, core narratives have been analysed through a psychoanalytic lens, allowing this approach to emerge within the data. Trauma has been depicted as the loss of life as we know it, which may trigger a core traumatic experience rooted in early years of life, the mother–infant relationship and eventual separation (Klein, 1952). Such a psychoanalytic perspective further enabled the multi-level analysis of data while explaining the way in which past events or experiences may have influenced individuals in the present, and especially in the way they face the consequences of the April 2020 lockdown measures including social distancing and isolation. In this way, it became possible to reveal the interplay between the effects of social circumstances and the struggles of the subject (participants) as they seek to position themselves in relation to themselves (Frosh et al., 2003).

Limitations

The sample of this study was collected during the first major lockdown, and since this occasion several developments have taken place (additional lockdowns, vaccination, new variants). Thus, a different timing might have offered different findings, and in that respect a repeated data collection might have proven fruitful; similarly, a comparative approach including data collected within different cultural settings might have offered more generalisable outcomes; however, the capacity of this study had been limited.

However, the limitation associated with the Greek focus of this study can become an advantageous starting point of future research as the structure of this data model is easily adaptable to other nationalities where the demographic is concentrated in the mother country but with nationals living in many other countries (Ireland, Israel, Albania etc.). Maintaining national homogeneity among participants residing in different parts of the world offers the unique opportunity to consider the ones living in the places other than homeland as a 'control group' by exploring whether they react similarly or along their peers in the homeland. In this way, one can see whether national identity is strengthened or not.

References

Alvesson, M. (2002). *Postmodernism and Social Research*. Open University Press.

Baker, C. (1997). Membership Categorisation and Interview Accounts. In D. Silverman (Ed.), *Qualitative Research*. Sage.

Becker, H. S. (1963). *Outsiders: Studies in the Sociology of Deviance*. Free Press.

BSA. (2022). *Guidelines on Ethical Research,* British Sociological Association. https://www.britsoc.co.uk/ethics

Charmaz, K., & Belgrave, L. L. (2015). Grounded Theory. In G. Ritzer (Ed.), *The Blackwell Encyclopedia of Sociology*. John Wiley & Sons.

Esterberg, K. G. (2002). *Qualitative Methods in Social Research*. McGraw Hill.

Frosh, S. (2010). *Psychoanalysis Outside the Clinic: Interventions in Psychosocial Studies*. Palgrave Macmillan.

Frosh, S., & Emerson, P. (2004). *Interpretation and Over-interpretation: Disrupting the Meaning of Texts in Qualitative Research, 5*(3), 307–324.

Frosh, S., Phoenix, A., & Pattman, R. (2003). Taking a Stand: Using psychoanalysis to Explore the Positioning of Subjects in Discourse. *British Journal of Social Psychology, 42*(1), 39–53. https://doi.org/10.1348/01446660 3763276117

Frosh, S., & Saville, Y. (2011). Psychoanalytic Approaches to Qualitative Psychology. In C. Willig & W. Stainton-Rogers (Eds.), *The SAGE Handbook of Qualitative Research in Psychology* (pp. 109–126). SAGE.

Gadamer, H.-G. (1976). *Philosophical Hermeneutics*. University of California Press.

Gadamer, H.-G. (2004). *Truth and Method*. Continuum Publishing Group.

Hoaglin, D., Mosteller, F., & Tukey, J. W. (1983). *Understanding Robust and Exploratory Data Analysis*. Wiley.

Hollway, W., & Jefferson, T. (2000). *Doing Qualitative Research Differently: Free Association Narrative and the Interview Method*. SAGE.

Jowett, A. (2021). Currying Out Qualitative Research under Lockdown-Practical and Ethical Considerations. *LSE Impact Block*. https://blogs.lse.ac.uk/impactof-socialsciences/2020/04/20/carrying-out-qualitative-research-under-lockdown-practical-and-ethical-considerations/

Klein, M. (1952). The Origins of Transference. *International Journal of Psychoanalysis, 33*, 433–438.

Kvale, S. (1996). *Inter Views: An Introduction to Qualitative Research Interviewing*. Sage.

Light, R. J., Singer, J., & Willet, J. (1990). *By Design: Conducting Research on Higher Education*. Harvard University Press.

Maxwell, J. A. (2013). *Qualitative Research Design: An Interactive Approach*. Sage.

Polit, D. F., & Beck, C. T. (2012). *Nursing Research: Generating and Assessing Evidence for Nursing Practice* (9th ed.).

Ricoeur, P. (1981/2016). *Hermeneutics and the Human Sciences: Essays on Language, Action, and Interpretation*. Cambridge University Press.

Ritchie, J., Lewis, J., McNaughton Nicholls, C., & Ormston, R. (Eds.). (2013). *Qualitative Research Practice. A Guide for Social Science Students and Researchers*. Sage.

Roseneil, S., & Budgeon, S. (2004). Cultures of Intimacy and Care beyond 'the Family': Personal Life and Social Change in the Early 21st Century. *Current Sociology, 52*(2), 135–159.

Ryan, G. W., & Bernard, H. R. (2003). Techniques to Identify Themes. *Field Methods, 15*(1), 85–109.

5

Experienced Change, Unsettlement and Crisis

Crisis and social change are two interrelated concepts sharing common ground as crisis is perceived as a transition which ultimately leads to social change (Koselleck & Richter, 2006). Gradual, as well as radical, transformation leads to an increase in uncertainty in people's lives in a number of different domains (Pinquart & Silbereisen, 2004) although radical social changes, like crises, are more related to unsettlement and disruption of continuity. In the first chapter, the Covid-19 pandemic had been discussed as a social change, causing transformations in both micro and macrosystems, taking the form of a disruptive and unsettling crisis. This chapter utilises this theoretical overview, to empirically analyse what this pandemic means to the participants of this study by focusing on the concepts of change and crisis. Participants' narratives have been primarily categorised into three types, following the theoretical approaches of the first chapter. The pandemic has been depicted as: (a) radical change involving lived transformations on macro and microsystems, (b) unsettlement and disruption and (c) crisis entailing fearful and hopeful perceptions.

Experienced Change

Approaching the Covid-19 pandemic as a social change enables us to realise that the effect of its radical and gradual transformations can be experienced through macro and microsystems as the pandemic has caused definite alterations on both collective and personal levels. Participants have experienced this pandemic on both levels through shared experiences of unforeseen social change, which has emerged suddenly and expanded rapidly, altering massively social and personal reality while challenging health, economic, political and social systems (Silbereisen, 2005). Participants narrated their experiences during the April 2020 lockdown through shared experiences of change which has affected various aspects of their everyday living. Some offered more macroscopic insights, by concentrating more on social, economic and political changes, whereas others were more concerned with the changes they experienced in their everyday lives.

(a) Change Experienced Through Macrosystems

According to Pinquart and Silbereisen (2004), transformations in macrosystems primarily concern transformations in society through changing laws or political and social institutions, and by new access to technical innovations. During the Coronavirus pandemic, governments around the world have implemented various methods of social restrictions in an attempt to reduce transmission (Harris et al., 2021); such measures causing significant alterations in everyday life can be perceived as alterations in the macrosystem. The following fragments reveal some of the participants' lived experiences of social, economic and political changes; Maria from Athens and Alina from London, for example, concentrate on the disastrous economic impact of this pandemic:

> Nothing will be as before. The economic crisis that emerges is huge and I am afraid that we will face serious economic impacts. (Maria, 68, Athens, retired, 2 kids)

> I view it as a huge change but I am not sure if it is for the better or worse. Financially will definitely be for the worse. (Alina, 40, London, married)

Sudden economic change and crisis is the main concern of the above participants and they both feel that the impact will be non-reversible and devastating, whereas Marina from London is also concerned about the future that such economic disaster may bring:

> I am very worried about what is going to happen next, how easily economies are going to fall apart and what kind of a world our children are going to live in. (Marina 40, London, employed, 2 kids)

Especially Marina's fragment reveals fearful concerns about the future of the economic collapse which will shape her children's life and thus entails long-lasting consequences. The common elements of the above fragments relate with the concerns of the participants relating to the consequences of the Covid-19 financial impact, which is inevitably related to a wider sense of uncertainty. Economic pressure has been identified as a distinct cause of distress (Goh et al., 2020) resulted from the transformation of economic systems whereas political implications are also involved. Eleni from Tokyo (Japan) and Theo from Northampton (UK) express their distress of the political changes and the impact on travelling:

> I feel [...] anger for some governments which allowed this situation to get out of control. I wanted to travel to Greece, but this was a reminder that maybe not everything is going as we desire. (Eleni, 29, Tokyo, suspended, married)

> The Greek government was the worst as denied the return of Greeks back to Greece. (Theo, 40, Northampton, student, in relationship)

The above fragments primarily reflect the anger of the participants towards governments who failed to confront Covid-19 effectively. Eleni and Theo share their distress of being unable to return to Greece, a feeling particularly vivid among diaspora Greeks. These fragments show that beyond the political impact of the governmental measures and policies, some participants felt prohibited from returning to their homeland; this particular prohibition is unprecedented as it expands beyond self-isolation measures adding isolation from one's homeland by the elimination of travelling. The prohibition of repatriation is not about the failure of governments to confront the pandemic but rather the denial of fundamental human rights in times of adversity resulting in a sense of abandonment. The desire to return home in adversity is an attachment-based and recuperative measure.

Economic, political and social transformations (gradual or radical) bring uncertainty in people's lives in a number of different domains (Pinquart & Silbereisen, 2004); Panos from Athens explains aspects of the social impact related to media and social contradictions related to ongoing social inequalities which have been particularly exposed during the pandemic (Grasso et al., 2020).

> There is a massive attempt by the media to misinform us, to turn our attention to minor issues whereas people die. This makes me feel tension. Many social contradictions have now become obvious like the abandonment of refugees vs the special treatment towards the Greek church. (Panos, 21, Athens, student, in relationship)

Social contradictions like the ones outlined above reflect deeper social inequalities which have become more obvious during the pandemic. As Tangjia (2014) explains crisis exposes the pre-existing symptoms of society and particularly serious remaining covered social problems including inequalities. Panos depicts the ways media reproduce such contradictions making him feel tension, or, from a psychoanalytic point of view, forcing one to become more conscious of social conflicts previously hidden. Such fragments reveal unforeseen sudden as well as potentially long-lasting alterations experienced on a macro-level, as have been perceived by the participants and related to Calhoun's (1992) depiction of social change as the process of alteration(s) of certain social characteristics such as social structures and institutions, norms, values, cultural products and symbols. Participants depicted the Covid-19 pandemic as a sudden albeit potentially enduring change in their political, economic and social environments affecting their future and the way they perceive their lives as they are primarily concerned about an impending economic catastrophe, which Greeks might be particularly sensitised too, and the ways governments have handled the pandemic and the social contradictions that have emerged.

More specifically, the above fragments depict fearful concerns and the uncertainty financial transformations have caused, whereas political measures and particularly the prohibition of repatriation have caused feelings of anger as it is associated with denial of fundamental human rights in times of adversity resulting in a sense of abandonment. Social inequalities have also been depicted as during times of crisis social contradictions may become more obvious causing tension.

Transformations on the macro-levels can cause rather personal reactions, and the impact of such transformations is experienced on a collective as well as on a personal level. At the same time, the Covid-19 pandemic has been depicted through lived transformations experienced on a micro-level, more related to everyday lives.

(b) Change Experienced Through Microsystems

The Covid-19 pandemic has also been experienced as a radical as well as a gradual transformation in microsystems, referring to the ways individuals relate to one another through alterations in family, school or workplace, that in turn affect the individual itself (Pinquart & Silbereisen, 2004). Such alterations have been experienced in several ways by the participants; for example, Kelly from Athens and Zenia from Crete (Greece) consider the lack of compassion and trust in human relations by stating that:

We should have been able to go through this crisis in a more collective way, but after all we only care about ourselves. (Kelly, 43, Athens, unemployed, 2 kids)

I feel that we need to take our personal responsibility to build a more qualitative world and focus on our actions […] However, instead of collaborating with each other and work collectively, we protect interests. And this makes me feel angry and produces uncertainty. I cannot trust that everything will go well since I have such thoughts. (Zenia, 38, Crete, employed, single)

As will be further discussed in the following chapter, human relations have been significantly affected by the pandemic in many respects, one of which relates with Kelly's and Zenia's concerns about individualistic attitudes as opposed to collective collaborations. In the above fragments there is a sense of disappointment because some people prioritise their own interests and Zenia expresses her consequent anger, distrust and uncertainty. Participants concentrated even further on human relations especially when referring to family and children. Parents, and particularly mothers, depicted sudden transformations in everyday life in relation to the way they needed to adjust, according to the needs of their children. Pratt (2020) maintains that families, individuals and social groups have had to develop coping strategies around caring for and schooling their children and employ creative combinations of demanding employed and parental roles within the context of isolation whereas gender inequalities have been revealed through such processes (Grasso et al., 2020). For example, Voula from Austria and Marina from London explain how they have managed to work and take care of their children during the lockdown:

> I have a three-year-old at home, so me and my husband have adjusted our programmes according to our child's needs. So we have divided the day to two shifts so that we can both work and take care of the kid. (Voula, 42, Austria, employed, married, 1 kid)

> I work from home, but I have changed the hours that I work so that I can take care of my kids during the day and work at night. (Marina, 40, London, employed, married, 2 kids)

Voula describes the radical adjustments that were needed in her family and everyday living in order to accommodate the needs of her child, and similarly, Marina explains that she had to work from home during night time in order to be able to take care of her children at home during the day. Kelly from Athens and Mari from Hong Kong explain how intensively their life has changed because their children can't go to school:

> My whole life has changed. Because I have a child who has stopped going to school so my everyday life has now changed. (Kelly, 43, Athens, unemployed, divorced, 2 kids)

The greatest difference is that my daughter used to go to school but not anymore. So I have to spend the whole day with her as my husband works long hours. I have no time for myself any more. (Mari, 40, Hong Kong, housewife, 1 kid, married)

As will be discussed in the next chapter, cohabitation became a new unsettling reality during lockdown, but in this case, the impact on mothers seems particularly intense. Although Kelly and Mari are not working, they explain how much their lives have changed because their children have stopped going to school. Being mothers entail the expectation that they should adjust their own lives in order to accommodate the needs of their children, which during the lockdown resulted in a lack of personal time and space. An additional aspect of gradual social change has to do with the use of online learning which has created a new reality utilised in all levels of education (Oosterhoff et al., 2020) resulting in increased reliance on digital technologies to enable some continuity of social and working lives (Pratt, 2020). Koralia from Bahrein shares her concerns about the new virtual reality her family experiences every day at home,

Now everything is virtual! Every day we begin with the online schooling. Then I will have to cook and play with them and then they will study again online. When my kids were going to school their mood was better. (Koralia, 40, Bahrein, housewife, 3 kids, married)

Koralia describes the way she accommodates and coordinates the online schooling routines of her three children while expressing her concern about the insufficiency of this alternative as her children were in a better mood before. Thus, Koralia not only spends the whole day taking care of her children's needs, but she is also concerned about their well-being because of the new digital realities. Kostas focuses on the transformed virtual contact he now experiences with his children:

My life has changed because everything is done through internet. Whenever I wanted to see my kids I could just visit them whereas now I can only see them through the screen. Technology has taken over. (Kostas, 60, Athens, employed, 2 kids, divorced)

Kostas describes the impact of technology on his life, which has enabled him to maintain contact with his children during lockdown, but at the same time he expresses his frustration as this contact is insufficient due to lack of physical proximity and ultimately lack of touch. In accordance with relevant literature, lockdown resulted in a general, pronounced decrease in family satisfaction, emergent lack of personal spaces, the complex management of different social roles and the collapse of the traditional boundaries between professional and private life (Möhring et al., 2020; Risi et al., 2020). Women specifically have been globally affected more as they still offer the largest part of unpaid work (Battyany, 2020), and they have been the main ones to combine housework, childcare and work-from-home activities (Collins et al., 2020; Möhring et al., 2020; Risi et al., 2020). The above fragments depict how everyday life has changed radically as well as gradually, because of the lockdown in relation to human relations and especially for families.

The above fragments also depict change as experienced through microsystems, including the concern about the individualistic rather than collective ways of dealing with the pandemic which reveals a sense of disappointment, anger, distrust and uncertainty. Notably, sudden and rather radical collective transformations have been depicted particularly in relation to family life of those having underaged children. Participants (primarily mothers) voiced shared transformations in the routines of everyday life as they narrated the radical adaptations needed to combine working from home and taking care of their children, devoting all their personal time and space to family and online schooling while adjusting gradually to a digital daily life which has replaced school and physical contact. Motherhood in particular entails the expectation that they should adjust their own lives in order to accommodate the needs of their children, which, during the lockdown, resulted in lack of personal time and space.

The lived experiences of participants reveal shared experiences of radical as well as gradual and ongoing change in both macro and microsystems entailing perceptions of political, social and economic changes as well as alterations in human relations, particularly within family life. Especially radical social changes have an impact on all aspects of human life including education (in this case online schooling), employment, family life and even leisure (Sennett, 1998). This radical change is quite commonly associated with Durkheim's state of 'anomie' (Durkheim, 1951/1897) while it is characterised by profound unsettlement. The following section expands further on human relations while being effected by disruption and unsettlement.

Unsettlement and Disruption

As will be further maintained in the following chapter, lived experiences of social isolation during the measures of April 2020 lockdowns have been depicted primarily through unsettlement and disruption. According to the relevant literature, change and crisis are interrelated and characterised by disruption of time, as well as the fragility and instability of the current (Hall, 2019). In the context of the Covid-19 pandemic, the distinct measure of self-isolation during lockdowns has formed a rather unique unsettlement and disruption of continuity, affecting personal as well as social life (Brooks et al., 2020). Disruption and unsettlement have been experienced in various ways by the participants; some participants, like Andreas from Belgium, depict the aspect of discontinuity in daily routines:

> It's a big change as the belief we had that we live in an unchangeable routine has been permanently disrupted. (Andreas, 27, Belgium, student, single)

And similarly, Mari from Hong Kong depicts the disruption of planning as:

> an overthrow of whatever we thought was given. Everything we have planned is up in the air particularly for those of us living away from home. (Mari, 40, Hong, Kong, housewife, 1 kid, married)

The above fragments portray a sudden transformation in daily lives which has left participants surprised and perhaps even cornered as the lack of prior relevant experience reinforces a sense of uncertainty. In the same vein, the disruption caused by the impact of the lockdown measures in particular has been portrayed as entailing loss of freedom and interruption of daily routines (Bao et al., 2020; Duan & Zhu, 2020) as narrated by Kiki from Athens:

> I feel imprisoned. I am not able to go out any more to meet friends to talk with other human beings. (Kiki, 32, Athens, single, employed)

Kiki expresses the difficulty of her experienced quarantine while characterising it as 'imprisonment' implying that the inability to get in contact with others due to the lockdown measures is equivalent to isolation experienced in prison. Such depicted daily realities portray the impact of the elimination of social contacts (Best et al. 2020) causing a tremendous effect on mental health on both personal and collective levels (Cardenas et al., 2020) as explained by Alex from Copenhagen:

> It means living my life by spending endless hours at home unable to socialise in a physical way. (Alex, 28, Copenhagen, employed, single)

For Alex, the way he is living his life has been restricted within the walls of his home, thus prohibiting physical socialisation; this fragment emphasises the significance of socialisation in the conceptualisation of what it means for a human being to live his/her life. The need to refer explicitly to a life without socialisation denotes an incomplete life. The lockdown periods, like that in April 2020 experienced by the participants, have been depicted in the literature as entailing fear, frustration and boredom (Brooks et al., 2020) exactly as described by Nikos from Eindhoven and Achilleas from Athens:

> For me this is a very boring, dead period which will eventually determine everyone's future. (Nikos, 26, Eindhoven, employed, single)

> I haven't left home for 30 or 40 days, but it is for a good cause so I can take it. But I feel very sad for humanity for all these deaths. (Achilleas, 58, Athens, employed, single)

Both Nikos and Achilleas depict the lockdown period as lost time while spending long days indoors without providing any details of how days are spent. Such omission entails a sense of 'dead time' as Nikos mentioned, lacking content or even meaning. Thus, lockdown is depicted as a period of time which has not been lived. Social isolation may even lead to personal and social uncertainty and loss of control (Brooks et al., 2020) also described by Evi from Athens:

> Everything is very odd because we have locked ourselves indoors, not knowing what to do with so much time in our hands while the crisis is killing people. It's really awkward. (Evi, 21, Athens, student, single)

Like Nikos and Achilleas, Evi feels unable to use the quarantine time in specific ways or to produce a course of action. Once again, there is a sense of participants feeling cornered or even trapped while feeling unable to react. This gives the impression of feeling immobilised due to uncertainty rather than danger. For some participants, the impact of the pandemic's disruption and unsettlement was more profound than others, and perhaps more related to a sense of fear, uncertainty (Gori & Topino, 2021; Ren et al., 2020; Wang et al., 2020), loneliness, psychosocial distress and lower levels of life satisfaction (Benke et al., 2020). For example, a profound level of distress is revealed by Elena from Athens:

> Because of the Greek crisis I remained unemployed and ultimately depressed for many years. Once things started to improve it was the turn of pandemic. So for me it was one crash after the other. All my dreams and prospects, once again, have fallen apart. (Elena, 35, Athens, employed, expecting)

Contrary to the previous fragments, Elena is voicing a depressed rather than immobilised attitude. She explains how damaging this pandemic has been for her since she experiences it as the extension of the prior painful Greek crisis which has caused her additional agony. It is thus seen that change in terms of unsettlement and disruption has been depicted by the participants primarily through shared experiences of social isolation due to lockdown. Although different participants depicted unsettlement and disruption in different ways, there is a consensus that no matter the geographical area they have found themselves in, social isolation has been a core part of their lived experiences of the Covid-19 pandemic. In line with the relevant literature, shared lived experiences of social isolation include disruption and unsettlement in daily routines, planning and travelling, loss of freedom, elimination of social contacts, boredom, frustration and loss of control as well as loneliness and distress.

More specifically, the participants of this section voiced additional aspects of unsettlement and disruption through feelings of being uncertain, surprised and perhaps even cornered. Quarantine has been depicted as equivalent to isolation experienced in prison whereas a life without socialisation denotes an incomplete life entailing 'dead time' as the lockdown period has been depicted as a period of time which has not been lived. Some participants even gave the impression of being immobilised due to uncertainty whereas expressed depression has also been revealed. Those components portray the participants' depiction of lockdown as a collective experience of change through unsettlement and disruption of continuity.

Fuchs (2020) uses the term "corona crisis" to describe the fact that social reality has been interrupted and altered during the pandemic whereas routines and everyday practices were completely reorganised. Notably, participants used the term change in its various contexts as well as the term crisis to refer to the Covid-19 pandemic, in their attempt to depict the ways that have experienced such radical social change on both collective and personal levels.

Experienced Crisis

The notion of crisis has been used repeatedly in everyday language to refer to the Covid-19 pandemic along with the concept of change. The participants of this study used these terms in various contexts in order to depict what the pandemic means to them. Matthewman and Huppatz (2020) explain that disasters, like Covid-19, are essentially social phenomena, and consequent threats and experiences are public and shared. The Covid-19 pandemic has been depicted by participants as a shared crisis, entailing a plurality of components aligned with relevant literature and initially related with danger and fear (Koselleck & Richter, 2006) followed by the aspects of opportunity and hope (French et al., 2009). This section reveals the two sides of crisis as narrated through the lived experiences of the participants.

(a) Fearful and Dangerous

Commonly, the meaning of crisis has been connected with the danger which is supposed to coexist with fear and uncertainty (Tangjia, 2014). In this vein, Ward (2020) explains that Covid-19 is primarily related to concepts of risk, fear, panic and lack of trust as well as individualisation, isolation and uncertainty. As already seen in previous sections, those concepts have been dominant in participants' narratives, whereas the following fragments approach the same concepts in different ways; for example, some participants perceived the pandemic as a global crisis entailing the elements of vulnerability. Argiro from Reykjavik explains:

> It's a crisis that showed us how vulnerable humans are. We give all of our time thinking about the pettiness of our daily routines and we forget how fragile life is. (Argiro, 40, Reykjavik, subsidised, married)

The pandemic is depicted as crisis by Argiro, which is signified as vulnerability through the risk of losing one's life because of Covid-19; this vulnerability overshadows the trivial insignificance of daily routines and becomes a priority. For Mary from Crete (Greece) this crisis is about panic and uncertainty:

> Panic from one day to the next. This crisis started very far away and now it's everywhere. I am trying not to let myself feel sadness and panic, although uncertainly is my main concern. (Mary, 66, Crete, retired, 2 kids, married)

Mary associates Covid-19 with a crisis which has expanded rapidly, spreading panic, sadness and uncertainty; Maria seems surprised, if not shocked, while trying to prevent these feelings overwhelm her. In the same vein, Thanos from Kastoria (Greece) refers to fear:

This crisis is all about being able to control our fear. Nothing else can help. Whatever is meant to happen will happen. (Thanos, 36, Kastoria, employed, single)

For Thanos, the Covid-19 crisis is conceptualised through fear which humans need to control as we are unable to do anything other than that. This fragment depicts this crisis through fear by acknowledging the incapability of humans to produce any form of viable action; at the same time though it implies a way to empowerment, through controlling our fears. Thus, through the conceptualisation of crisis as fear (instead of danger and disaster) humans can actually do something, by controlling their own fears, and consequently controlling the crisis. Fear and panic have certainly been fundamental components of the Covid-19 pandemic which have been reported as "Covid-19 phobia" (Lindinger-Sternart et al., 2021) and "coronaphobia" (Asmundson & Taylor, 2020; Brooks et al., 2020) denoting the vulnerability and insecurity associated to the fear of potential infection. An additional way that the crisis of Covid-19 has been depicted is as a human crisis as noted by Iason from Copenhagen:

It is a human crisis apart from the health crisis. We could have been more prepared; we had seen evidence that something like that may happen. (Iason, 28, Copenhagen, unemployed, single)

The human crisis for Iason means that humanity was unprepared to confront Covid-19 although it should have been able to do so. Therefore, Iason implies that something must have gone wrong as humans are not able to collectively protect themselves from the danger of the pandemic. Thus, crisis is more related to failure of being collectively protected in this context. A similar context of crisis can be seen through the form of distrust towards governments, statistics, science, media, technology (Calnan, 2020) and political institutions (Risi et al., 2020). Such reactions are more related to distrust as this crisis has been ineffectively managed. Distrust has also been depicted towards other people (Ward, 2020), as very characteristically portrayed by Theo from Northampton (UK):

This crisis has let lots of our ugliness to be seen. People caring for themselves, emptying supermarkets, behaving on a survival mode. (Theo, 40,
Northampton, student, in relationship)

Theo associates the Covid-19 crisis with ugliness deriving from individualistic rather than collective reactions, a concern depicted previously
by Kelly and Zenia. Thus, crisis here is related to Iason's view of a pre-
pandemic human crisis again associated with failure, but in this case it
was the failure of acting collectively in a more humanitarian way whereas
Iason was referring to the failure of being collectively prepared to protect
ourselves from this pandemic.

In line with the primary depiction of crisis through fear and danger
(Koselleck & Richter, 2006), participants have used such characteristics
to portray their own understanding and experience of the pandemic,
which again seems to be unrelated to the geographical areas in which
participants reside. Lived experiences of crises ultimately become manifestations of life crisis shaping life course, biographies and imaginaries of
the future. In that sense, economic, political or social crises convert to
personal crises (Hall, 2019). Indeed, participants depicted Covid-19 as a
crisis entailing vulnerability primarily related to public health; it has been
described as a crisis which has expanded rapidly, entailing panic, sadness
and uncertainty while at the same time it has been conceptualised through
fear (rather than danger or destruction) albeit aiming at empowerment
through controlling the crisis while controlling our fears. The Covid-19
crisis has also been depicted through failure to collectively act in a
humanitarian way, as well as the failure of being prepared and able to
protect ourselves from this pandemic. Thus, crisis may be perceived in
different ways depending on how people conceptualise and experience it.

Notably, there are two sides in each crisis as it can be experienced as
both danger and an opportunity (Tangjia, 2014) because crises entail
change as well as opportunities to impose new ideas and practices (French
et al., 2009). This side of the crisis has been revealed by several participants offering an additional perspective on the lived experiences of the
pandemic.

(b) Opportunity for Improvement

Silbereisen et al. (2006) maintain that individuals are neither passive recipients nor victims of social change, and most of them cope actively with social change, whereas Hall (2019) adds that crises can offer possibilities for change and continuity. Such perspectives have been incorporated by several participants like Giannis from Tokyo Koralia from Bahrein and Lia from Brussels who have depicted the aspect of positive opportunity within the Covid-19 context:

> This pandemic for me means half challenge and half opportunity. (Giannis, 59, Tokyo, employed, 1 kid, married)

> It's like a restart, an opportunity to re-evaluate whatever we thought given. (Koralia, 40, Bahrein, housewife, 3 kids, married)

> We can re-evaluate circumstances both in governmental and individual levels. We realise what is important to us and what is not. We can also make good use of it and become better as individuals and states or not. (Lia, 28, Brussels, employed, single)

Giannis (Tokyo) depicts the pandemic both as a challenge and as an opportunity, while Koralia (Bahrein) perceives it as an opportunity to re-evaluate whatever we have been relying on. In similar ways, Lia (Brussels) views the opportunity to evaluate what is important on a personal and national level and act accordingly. Thus, the crisis can be perceived as an opportunity to improve. Indeed, Tangjia (2014) explains that people who can recognise opportunity in crisis are those with a clear awareness of what is happening and can successfully find a safe way through it, like Natalia from the UK and Aggelos from the USA who display self-awareness and self-support:

> It's a good lesson that we need to learn. To become stronger and move on although no one was prepared for a crisis like that. (Natalia, 29, Northampton, suspended, in relationship)

> For me it's a gift of time, a 'pause' that each one of us can use constructively or simply let it go. It's a great opportunity to prove ourselves that we can handle this crisis. (Aggelos, 23, Los Angeles, part-time employed, single)

Natalia's fragment depicts this crisis as a lesson teaching us how to be stronger and move on although people have not been prepared to confront this crisis; similarly, Aggelos narrate the crisis as a gift of additional time (in contradiction to previous depiction of lockdowns as 'dead time') offering the opportunity to make good use of it by overcoming the crisis. Although neither Natalia nor Aggelos explain how they plan to utilise the opportunity to overcome this crisis, they both display a rather positive and optimistic attitude which can be proved helpful and self-supportive. According to Home (2020) and Neal (1998), disruptive events may also offer new opportunities for innovation and change; crises and radical social change do not only cause worry and fear but also anticipation and hope (Tangjia, 2014) as they can offer possibilities for change and continuity while forming lived, intimate and very personal experiences (Hall, 2019). Aggeliki and Aris from Athens reveal their own lived experiences through appreciating what they have, being aware of themselves and the situation they experience while becoming self-supportive.

> It's a 'pause' so that we can see what is going on inside us and around us. Once the time will come to press 'play' again, then we can decide if our life is as we want it to be if the people around us are the ones we want. (Aggeliki, 46, Athens, employed, expecting, in relationship)

> This pandemic for me means a gift of extra time added to a crazy and demanding everyday life, to reflect upon my life, my family, my work, my friends. I am happy for that. (Aris, 42, Athens, employed, 1 kid, married)

Aggeliki perceives the pandemic as a 'pause', as a time discontinuity which can be used for introspection and evaluation of ourselves and others. Slowing down time gives the opportunity to consider what works in one's life and what should change; thus, Aggeliki focuses on a constructive utilisation of her time, while supporting herself through this opportunity. Similarly, Aris explains that he feels happy for being able to slow down his demanding routine and be able to reflect upon his life. Both fragments reveal ways that Aggeliki and Aris have employed to support themselves constructively. Additionally, Lazarus and Folkman (1984) explain that coping strategies include trying to change the problem that is causing the distress, and Bacevic and McGoey (2021) maintain that during the Covid-19 pandemic people's capacity for adaption, reflection and social organisation has been evident as seen through the examples of Lia from Belgium and Nora from Athens who have focused on self-improvement and self-help:

> I see the chance to reconsider everything really and the opportunity to become better humans instead of falling apart. (Lia, 28, Belgium, employed, single)

> I don't feel helpless, alone or desperate. I have started adjusting my every-day life to this lockdown. It's something imposed to all of us, it won't last forever and eventually we will get out of it. We are all in the exact same situation globally. But I am hopeful, we will make it. (Nora, 42, Athens, employed, single)

Like Aggeliki and Aris, Lia (Belgium) describes an opportunity to improve ourselves through self-awareness while Nora (Athens) becomes more specific in describing that what makes her hopeful is the realisation that all humans go through the same experience and that this will pass too. For Tangjia (2014), there is no better way to overcome a crisis than sympathetic understanding, considerate care and mutual help. Coping strategies that have been proven helpful during the pandemic have been identified by relevant literature include seeking social support and positive thinking (Anwar et al., 2020). Such attitudes can be seen through the examples of Bill from the USA and Kostas from Athens who reveal kindness, empathy, self-awareness and self-support as follows:

> It's all about taking care of ourselves and the people next to us. (Bill, 78, Maryland, retired, married)

> Although I feel that I am running out of energy, I don't feel angry. This pandemic is about testing relationships of all kinds. The stronger ones will survive the others will fall apart. Especially if you are locked under the same roof! Understanding, respect, lots of love and a bit of humour is needed to get pass this. And I know that we will make it. (Kostas, 60, Athens, employed, 2 kids, divorced)

Bill acknowledges the significance of empathy and caring towards others as well as oneself while Kostas becomes self-aware while evaluating his own feelings. He refers to family cohabitation during quarantine (also discussed in the following chapter) which, although it can prove challenging, can be managed through understanding, respect, love and humour. Notably, there are people who not only survive challenging circumstances but they become strengthened by the particular exposure to adversity; according to Papadopoulos (2004, 2006), positive developments are possible as direct results of being exposed to adversity. Voula's example demonstrates this exact case by appreciating what she has while supporting and rewarding herself. She says:

> This pandemic for me was like vacation because I was very lucky. Because I didn't lose my job permanently, I didn't have to work and take care of my children within a small flat all day long, I didn't have a vulnerable member of my family to protect. All I had to do is lock myself indoors, fill up my fridge and let the time pass. I wouldn't have said the same if I was working long shifts at a supermarket while being a parent. (Voula, 42, Austria, suspended, 1 kid, married)

The reflexive fragment of Voula (from Austria) reveals her willingness and ability to concentrate on the aspects of her life about which she feels grateful, like the fact that she is still employed (although suspended); this has given her the opportunity to take care of her kid, the fact that she does not have to protect a vulnerable member of her family, that she is able to fill up her fridge and just be patient. Voula acknowledges that her life situation would have been very different if she had to work at a supermarket while being a parent. This narrative reflects gratitude and an ability to become self-supportive as a means employed by Voula to cope with this pandemic.

Pratt (2020) maintains that the unfamiliarity of 'lockdown' has been a challenge to our societies and the ways we care for others. Families, individuals and social groups have had to develop coping strategies of caring and schooling and employ creative combinations of demanding roles within the context of isolation. Crisis has indeed two sides, and the analysed fragments of this section revealed that the Covid-19 pandemic is no exception. Although crisis often appears suddenly and people do not have enough time to react and take action, we can nevertheless work out some plans to cope with crisis ahead of time by putting positive and useful elements into full use to eliminate crisis (Tangjia, 2014).

Participants of this section have depicted the Covid-19 pandemic primarily as an opportunity to improve matters mainly on a personal level. They became more specific about the ways that they have employed to achieve that: by evaluating what is important and act accordingly; remaining positive and optimistic; being aware of themselves and the situation they experience; utilising time constructively; being hopeful through the realisation that all humans go through the same experience and that this will pass too; through empathy and caring towards others as well as oneself; through understanding, respect, love and humour; and finally through gratitude of what they have and willingness to become and remain self-supportive. Ultimately, portraying crisis as opportunity rather than fear enabled participants to concentrate on means employed to cope with the pandemic.

Synopsis

This chapter analysed the participants' lived experiences of the Covid-19 pandemic by concentrating on their depiction of Covid-19 primarily through the concepts of change, unsettlement and disruption as well as crisis. Based on the relevant literature, shared experiences among participants associated with the April 2020 lockdown entail meaning-making of the pandemic in terms of (a) experienced change in both macro and microsystems, (b) experienced unsettlement and disruption and finally (c) experienced crisis as fear and danger as well as opportunity for improvement. These categories have allowed for a synthesised mosaic to emerge in terms of how different people, residing in different places in the world, have created meaning-making of their shared experience during the April 2020 lockdown. This mosaic offered the opportunity to synthesise a rich plurality of shared experiences, shining a light on the meaning-making of this pandemic.

Based on the participants' narratives, the Covid-19 pandemic entailed the following distinct shared experiences:

(a) In terms of change through *macrosystems*, participants depicted the Covid-19 pandemic as a sudden change in their political, economic and social environments. More specifically, participants have voiced fearful concerns about the uncertainty financial transformations have caused; anger towards political measures and particularly the prohibition of repatriation resulting in a sense of abandonment; tension caused by the intensification of social inequalities and contradictions.

Change has also been depicted through *microsystems*, entailing shared feelings of disappointment, anger, distrust and uncertainty associated with the individualistic rather than collective ways of dealing with the pandemic, whereas parents (primarily mothers) narrated the ways they have adjusted and devoted their personal time and space to their families and online schooling while working from home, taking care of their children and adjusting to a digital daily life which has replaced school and physical contact.

(b) Regarding shared lived experiences of unsettlement and disruption during the April 2020 lockdowns, the participants voiced shared feelings of being: surprised, cornered, depressed, imprisoned and even immobilised because of uncertainty. There was a sense that life without socialisation denotes an incomplete life and that the lockdown period is a period of time which has not been lived entailing 'dead time'.

(c) In relation to the concept of crisis, participants depicted Covid-19 as a crisis which has expanded rapidly, entailing panic, sadness, vulnerability and uncertainty while at the same time it has been conceptualised through fear albeit aiming at empowerment through controlling the crisis while controlling our fears. The Covid-19 crisis has also been depicted through failure to collectively act in a humanitarian way, as well as a failure of being prepared and able to protect ourselves from this pandemic. Portraying crisis through fear prohibited participants from forming coping strategies.

At the same time the pandemic has been portrayed as a crisis offering an opportunity for improvement by evaluating what is important and acting accordingly; remaining positive and optimistic; being aware of oneself and the external situation; utilising time constructively; being hopeful through the realisation that all humans go through the same experience and that this will pass too; through empathy and caring towards others as well as oneself; through understanding, respect, love and humour. Finally, this opportunity for improvement was portrayed through gratitude for what we have and willingness to become and remain self-supportive. Ultimately, portraying crisis as an opportunity rather than fear enabled participants to concentrate on the different ways to cope with the pandemic.

Bibliography

Anwar, A., Malik, M., Raees, V., & Anwar, A. (2020). Role of Mass Media and Public Health Communications in the COVID-19 Pandemic. *Cureus, 12*, e10453–e10453.

Asmundson, G. J. G., & Taylor, S. (2020). Coronaphobia: Fear of the 2019-nCoV Outbreak. *Journal of Anxiety Disorders, 70*, 102196.

Bao, Y., Sun, Y., Meng, S., Shi, J., & Lu, L. (2020). 2019-nCoV Epidemic: Address Mental Health Care to Empower Society. *Lancet, 395*(10224), e37–e38.

Bacevic, J. and McGoey, L., (2021). *Surfing Ignorance: Covid-19 and the Rise of Fatalistic Liberalism, Research Repository*. University of Essex (Unpublished). http://repository.essex.ac.uk/30721/

Battyany, K. (2020). The Covid-19 Pandemic Reveals and Exacerbates the Crisis of Care. *Open Democracy*. https://www.opendemocracy.net/en/openmovements/covid-19-pandemic-reveals-and-exacerbates-crisis-care/

Benke, C., Autenrieth, L. K., Asselmann, E., & Pané-Farré, C. A. (2020). Lockdown, Quarantine Measures, and Social Distancing: Associations with Depression, Anxiety and Distress at the Beginning of the COVID-19 Pandemic among Adults from Germany. *Psychiatry Research, 293*, 113462.

Best, L. A., Law, M. A., Roach, S., & Wilbiks, J. M. P. (2020). The Psychological Impact of COVID-19 in Canada: Effects of Social Isolation During the Initial Response. *Canadian Psychology*. https://doi.org/10.1037/cap0000254

Brooks, S. K., Webster, R. K., Smith, L. E., Woodland, L., Wessely, S., Greenberg, N., & Rubin, G. J. (2020). The Psychological Impact of Quarantine and How to Reduce It: Rapid Review of the Evidence. *Lancet, 395*(10227), 912–920.

Calhoun, C. (1992). Social Change. In E. F. Borgatta & M. L. Borgatta (Eds.), *Encyclopedia of Sociology* (Vol. 4, pp. 1807–1812). Macmillan.

Calnan, M. (2020). Health Policy and Controlling Covid-19 in England: Sociological Insights. *Emerald Open Research, 2*(40), 2–14. https://doi.org/10.35241/emeraldopenres.13726.2

Cardenas, M. C., Bustos, S. S., & Chakraborty, R. (2020). A 'parallel pandemic': The Psychosocial Burden of COVID-19 in Children and Adolescents. *Acta pædiatrica, 109*(11), 2187–2188.

Collins, C., Landivar, L. C., Ruppanner, L., & Scarborough, W. J. (2020). COVID-19 and the Gender Gap in Work Hours. *Gender, Work & Organization*. https://doi.org/10.1111/gwao.12506.

Duan, L., & Zhu, G. (2020). Psychological Interventions for People Affected by the COVID-19 Epidemic. *Lancet Psychiatry, 7*(4), 300–302.

Durkheim E. (1951[1897]). *Suicide: A Study in Sociology* (J. A. Spaulding, & G. Simpson, Trans.). The Free Press.

French, S., Leyshon, A., & Thrift, N. (2009). A Very Geographical Crisis: The Making and Breaking of the 2007–2008 Financial Crisis. *Cambridge Journal of Regions, Economy and Society, 2*(2), 287–302.

Fuchs, C. (2020). 'Everyday Life and Everyday Communication in Coronavirus Capitalism', Triple C: Communication, Capitalism & Critique. *Open Access Journal for a Global Sustainable Information Society, 18*(1), 375–398.

Goh, K. K., Lu, M. L., & Jou, S. (2020). 'Impact of COVID-19 Pandemic: Social Distancing and the Vulnerability to Domestic Violence. *Psychiatry and Clinical Neurosciences, 74*(11), 612–613.

Gori, A., & Topino, E. (2021). Across the COVID-19 Waves—Assessing Temporal Fluctuations in Perceived Stress, Post-traumatic Symptoms, Worry, Anxiety and Civic Moral Disengagement Over one year of Pandemic. *International Journal of Environmental Research and Public Health, 18*(11), 5651.

Grasso, M., Klicperová-Baker, M., Koos, S., Kosyakova, Y., Petrillo, A., & Vlase, I. (2020). The Impact of the Coronavirus Crisis on European Societies., What Have we Learned and Where Do We Go from Here? Introduction to the Covid Volume. *European Societies., 23*(S1), 2–32.

Hall, S. M. (2019). A Very Personal Crisis: Family Fragilities and Everyday Conjunctures Within Lived Experiences of Austerity. *Transactions of the Institute of British Geographers, 44,* 479–492.

Harris, D.; Ellis, D. Y, , Gorman, D.; Foo, N, and Haustead, D. (2021) 'Impact of COVID-19 Social Restrictions on Trauma Presentations in South Australia' *Emergency Medicine AUSTRALASIA, 33* (1): 152–154

Home. (2020, July). Collective Trauma Amid Covid: Excerpt from 'Together Apart'. https://www.socialsciencespace.com/2020/07/collective-trauma-amid-covid-excerpt-from-together-apart/

Koselleck, R., & Richter, M. W. (2006). Crisis. *Journal of the History of Ideas, 67*(2), 357–400.

Lazarus R. S., & Folkman S. (1984). Stress, Appraisal and Coping. New York: Springer.

Lindinger-Sternart, S., Kaur, V., Widyaningsih, Y., & Patel, A. K. (2021). COVID-19 Phobia across the World: Impact of Resilience on COVID-19 Phobia in Different Nations. *Counselling and Psychotherapy Research, 21*(2), 290–302.

Matthewman, S., & Huppatz, K. (2020). A Sociology of Covid-19. *Journal of Sociology, 46*(4), 675–683.

Möhring, K., Naumann, E., Reifenscheid, M., Wenz, A., Rettig, T., Krieger, U., Friedel, S., Finkel, M., Cornesse, C., & Blom, A. G. (2020). The COVID-19 Pandemic and Subjective Well-being: longitudinal evidence on Satisfaction with Work and Family. *European Societies*, 1–17. https://doi.org/10.108 0/14616696.2020.1833066

Neal, A. G. (1998). *National Trauma and Collective Memory: Major Events in the American Century.* M. E. Sharpe, Armonk.

Oosterhoff, B., Palmer, C. A., Wilson, J., & Shook, N. (2020). Adolescents' Motivations to Engage in Social Distancing during the COVID-19 Pandemic: Associations with Mental and Social Health. *Journal of Adolescent Health, 67,* 179–185.

Papadopoulos, R. K. (2004). *Trauma in a Systemic Perspective: Theoretical, Organizational and Clinical Dimensions.* Paper presented at the 14th Congress of the International Family Therapy Association, Istanbul.

Papadopoulos, R. K. (2006). Terrorism and Panic. *Psychotherapy and Politics International, 4*(2), 90–100.

Pinquart, M., & Silbereisen, R. K. (2004). Human Development in Times of Social Change: Theoretical Considerations and Research Needs. *International Journal of Behavioral Development, 28,* 289–298.

Pratt, A. C. (2020). Covid-19 Impacts Cities, Cultures and Societies. *City, Culture and Society., 21*, 1–2.

Ren, S. Y., Gao, R. D., & Chen, Y. L. (2020). Fear Can Be More Harmful Than the Severe Acute Respiratory Syndrome Coronavirus 2 in Controlling the Coronavirus Disease 2019 Epidemic. *World Journal of Clinical Cases, 8*(4), 652–657.

Risi, E., Pronzato, R., & Fraia, G. (2020). Everything is Inside the Home: The Boundaries of Home Confinement During the Italian lockdown. *European Societies*, 1–14. https://doi.org/10.1080/14616696.2020.1828977

Sennett, D. (1998). *Der flexible Mensch: Die Kultur des neuen Kapitalismus [The Flexible Person: On the Culture of the New Capitalism]* (8th edn.). Berlin Verlag.

Silbereisen, R. K. (2005). Social Change and Human Development: Experiences from German Unification. *International Journal of Behavioral Development, 29*, 2–13.

Silbereisen, R. K., Pinquart, M., Reitzle, M., Tomasik, M. J., Fabel, K., & Grümer, S. (2006). Psychosocial Resources and Coping with Social Change. http://psydok.psycharchives.de/jspui/bitstream/20.500.11780/460/1/sfb_580_silbereisen_5.pdf

Tangjia, W. (2014, June). A Philosophical Analysis of the Concept of Crisis. *Frontiers of Philosophy in China, 9*(2), 254–267.

Wang, C., Pan, R., Wan, X., Tan, Y., Xu, L., Ho, C. S., & Ho, R. C. (2020). Immediate Psychological Responses and Associated Factors During the Initial Stage of the 2019 Coronavirus Disease (COVID-19) Epidemic among the General Population in China. *International Journal of Environmental Research and Public Health, 17*(5), 1729.

Ward, P. R. (2020). A Sociology of the Covid-19 Pandemic: A Commentary and Research Agenda for Sociologists. *Journal of Sociology*, 1–10. https://doi.org/10.1177/1440783320939682

6

Experienced Trauma Through Loss

Our understanding of trauma, confirmed by the literature review primarily associates it with fundamental experiences of loss (Klein, 1952, 1955). This chapter utilises relevant theoretical approaches in order to discuss the ways participants may have experienced traumatic aspects of Covid-19 in various domains of life that have been influenced by the April 2020 lockdowns and the consequent quarantine and social isolation measures. The thematic categories revealed in this section relate to consequences of trauma through: (a) symbiosis, (b) isolation and (c) disruption of time continuity. Trauma is also discussed as a collective experience which has been subsequently categorised through shared experiences of (a) denial of loss and (b) acceptance of loss. This chapter empirically analyses what this pandemic means to the participants of the study by focusing on trauma associated with various experiences of loss.

Experienced Trauma

According to Kalsched (2021, p. 444), trauma refers to the incidents that "we are all given more to experience in this life than we can bear to experience consciously". Considering the impact of the Covid-19 pandemic,

A. Chalari, E. E. Koutantou, *Psycho-Social Approaches to the Covid-19 Pandemic*,
https://doi.org/10.1007/978-3-031-07831-6_6

trauma can become an inevitable aspect of the Covid-19 pandemic for many people as life continuity has been significantly disrupted (Schejtman, 2021). This loss of life prior to the pandemic may trigger a core traumatic experience for some, rooted in the early years of life, the mother-infant relationship and eventual separation (Klein, 1952). In line with discussed psychoanalytic literature on trauma and the review on collective trauma, this chapter analyses participants' fragments in relation to traumatic experiences associated with April 2020 lockdown narratives and focuses on specific aspects of daily life which has now been extensively altered.

A. Experienced Symbiosis

The first thematic category focuses on aspects of symbiosis approached as an intrapsychic experience (Angel, 1967, 1972; Harrison, 1986) which can be used to define experiential states (Meissner, 1981). Symbiosis is revealed through the fragments of participants for whom relationships with family members living in the same house have been negatively influenced because of the compulsory proximity during the social isolation measures of lockdowns. At the same time, relations with other people outside the house became challenging. Thus, the aspect of closeness and symbiosis within families may entail fluctuation. Below, one can see different aspects of how the participants experience symbiosis while living 'together'; for example, Aris from Athens explains that families have come closer during lockdown:

> Concerning family relations, families have come closer suddenly and compulsorily, which creates both enjoyable and disturbing circumstances. But I also think that human relationships remain very important and they are the big disclosure within this crisis; either you quarrel or you spend a good time. (Aris, 42, Athens, employed, 1 kid)

Aris discusses a rather splitting situation of the good and bad aspects of what it means to come closer with family members living in the same house, perhaps related with Blass and Blatt's (1996) approach to symbiosis as 'merger' (in which two are experienced as joined together into one), whereas Antigoni explains a different, more optimistic view of this 'closeness', perhaps more related with approaches on symbiosis perceived as 'fusion' (in which the other is seen as part of oneself) (Nacht, 1964; Rose, 1964, 1972).

> My intimate relationships have been restricted. We can't meet each other. However, deep relationships became deeper and at the same time, the indifferent ones became stronger because we all share the same anxiety. Thus, this 'togetherness', the common experience we live can unite us more. (Antigoni, 60, Athens, suspended, single)

Both participants speak about the 'closeness' (and thus symbiosis) that emerged due to the quarantine, but in quite different ways. Antigoni glorifies the 'being together', claiming: "we all share the same anxiety", which can be traced back to the fear of losing care and love from our primordial objects (Freud, 1917). This shared fear 'will unite us' which reveals an experienced version of symbiosis more related to Meissner's (1981) perception of symbiosis as 'fusion'. Optimistic as it may seem, it may be based upon fear and uncertainty that such circumstances may generate, so it can collapse as soon as the measures are abolished. Aris, on the other hand, acknowledges the disturbing aspect of this 'closeness', which may be intensified due to the quarantine and related to Meissner's (1981) approach to symbiosis as 'merger'.

Social isolation measures may generate anxiety (Schejtman, 2021) which in turn results in bringing people closer to each other. In psychoanalytic words, anxiety originates from the fear of annihilation and of the unknown, a persecutory anxiety from inner sources that can become more intense when it meets painful external experience of frustration (Freud, A, 1936; Freud, S. 1920); the containing environment and the safety it provides, are then lost so the individual feels vulnerable and unprotected and being attacked from the bad external object (that is the environment, society, etc.) (Klein, 1946) or in this case Covid-19 pandemic.

Voula, from Austria, reinforces Aris' argument on 'closeness' while referring to families who cohabitate; this kind of symbiosis may entail unanticipated negative outcomes, including oppressed feelings:

Concerning our child, I think that he is very happy to spend more time with us so the relationship has become more intense and much more symbiotic [...]. I appreciate the fact that we can spend time together [with my child] but there are moments that I feel oppressed, because I have to play with him while I may feel bored. [...] In the beginning, it was difficult but now we have all found our rhythms and we like it. In the beginning, we were anxious with my husband [...]. We are a couple who discuss and negotiate about our boundaries and responsibilities and we try to ensure our space and time. (Voula, 42, Austria, suspended, 1 kid)

This fragment reflects the bright and the dark aspect of the symbiotic (Mahler et al., 1975) familial relationships as well as the bright and the dark aspect of motherhood during the quarantine from the perspective of the mother. Feelings of love and oppression are evident and the fear of losing oneself within the maternal role is clearly expressed. Such examples of prolonged and continuous cohabitation can generate oppression due to the compulsory daylong contact where there is no alternative. As discussed in the previous chapter, individuals in family (and particularly mothers) may exceed their boundaries, lose their personal space and time and merge with the other. In this case we refer to fear of symbiosis as 'fusion', as the lack of differentiation of self and the other (Meissner, 1981).

Zenia from Athens demonstrates this dimension from the perspective of the adult daughter, spending the lockdown with her parents in the same house:

We spend all the day with family and there are battles and nerves, which is expected because I spend a lot of time with them so this makes me crazy. I try to leave the house these moments to avoid conflict [...]. My friends experience the same with parents; we get angry with them very easily. (Zenia, 23, Athens, single, employed)

This fragment reveals the loss of personal space and time and this merge can drive individuals 'crazy', as Zenia claims. Zenia as a young adult needs to re-negotiate personal time and space while she re-lives her childish and teenage era again due to the prolonged cohabitation and the increasing getting in touch with parents. Zenia's experience may be associated with primary symbiosis (Pollock, 1964) in which one person attaches or clings to another person so both of them find a refuge for each other's unresolved needs.

Another aspect of symbiosis can be seen through the experience of 'closeness' expressed by participants who live abroad and claim that their relationships back in Greece have become closer while those formed in the country of their current residence have become worse, as discussed by Andreas from Brussels and Rita from Munich:

> On the one hand, the quarantine does not offer me the chance to socialise; on the other hand, I keep in touch with friends back in Greece via telephone and social media, something that I wouldn't do if a quarantine was not in place. I do not claim that this situation is fine but I assume that my relationships with people back in Greece have become better and more intense. However, my social life here has decreased a lot because I also work from home. (Andreas, 27, Brussels, single, student)

> Most of my contacts are in Greece and I had only a telephone contact with them anyway. It is so moving that people ask me if I am ok. My relationships have become better due to the circumstances. However, I miss people from the country of my current residence. And I miss the fact that I cannot travel back to Greece in this occasion. (Rita, 36, Munich, employed, single)

The examples above demonstrate that the need for contact due to the quarantine is intense for the Greek diaspora as well, but that the homeland serves as the familiar rather than their current country of residence. Of course, the quarantine measures restrict socialisation and human contact. Thus, the need for human contact is more intense with the family back in Greece, which, in psychoanalytic words, serves as the internal, good object, while the country of current residence serves as the external, bad object (Klein, 1932, 1935, 1946, 1952). There is a tendency to regress (Laplanche & Pontalis, 1981) to the internal, safe environment 'back' in the home country or 'motherland', even virtually. At this point, the country of residence serves as the foreigner that we are afraid of, as the other against whom one should be protected.

This sub-section discusses how symbiosis emerged due to the quarantine measures and social isolation. The term symbiosis is used to refer to the feature of primitive cognitive affective life wherein the differentiation between self and (m)other has not taken place or where regression (Freud,

1917) to that self-object undifferentiated state (which characterised the symbiotic phase) has recurred (Mahler et al., 1975). What remains significant though is the realisation that loss (experienced on this occasion through symbiosis) is associated with the meaning ascribed to it by each individual separately, consciously or unconsciously.

Different forms of experienced symbiosis have been depicted through participants' fragments who have to live under the same roof with family members and this experience has caused various fractions. Participants revealed that the compulsory proximity brings forced closeness making them feel oppressed whereas others have the tendency to merge with the other, mostly the family member with whom they cohabitate and especially with the parents. In times of crisis, regression back to the familiar and familial may act as the safe place that protects from potential anxiety. Fragments revealed challenging aspects of symbiosis entailing fusion and merger (as well as fear towards symbiosis), resulting in the loss of life as it was before the lockdown, loss of personal space and time. Additionally, primary symbiosis has also been revealed as a form of mutual coverage of respective needs between family members. Closeness (and lack of) has been depicted through narratives deriving particularly from the Greek diaspora emphasising the nostalgic need for contact with the homeland.

It is thus seen that external circumstances formed through the measures of social distancing and isolation forced people to distance from each other and remain indoors regardless of the region in which each participant resides. Individuals could not meet other people apart from family members living in the same house and could not continue outdoor activities, leisure activities, work outside and so forth. In turn, this condition forced many people to regress. Isolation and loneliness have been narrated by the participants as an additional consequential outcome of the above-mentioned measures employed during lockdowns in different parts of the world.

B. Isolation and Loneliness

As has already been identified in Chap. 5, significant effect of the self-isolation measure (as part of lockdowns) which has made relationships challenging is alienation from the other on a physical or an emotional level or even both. A significant number of participants feel isolated from their relatives, friends or families due to the lockdowns and the fear of the other as the potential carrier of the virus. At the same time, virtual contact is deemed insufficient. Psychosocial distress, including depression, can result from social isolation and quarantining (Jiao et al., 2020). In this vein, Giannis from Tokyo, Kelly from Athens and Bill from Baltimore share their own experienced isolations:

> Isolation is the biggest difficulty. (Giannis, 59, Tokyo, employed, 1 kid)

> Relationships are influenced because I have no contact with anybody [...]. They are influenced because we may not be in the mood to speak via phone anyway. (Kelly, 43, Athens, unemployed, divorced, 2 kids)

> Yes, relations have changed to the extent that we cannot have company at home and we cannot go to their places and we communicate only by phone or Skype. (Bill, 78, Maryland, retired, married)

Isolation as perceived by Klein (1975) and restriction in physical contact influence relationships and human contact. Thanos from Kastoria and Mary from Heraklion (Greece) express their discontent, sadness and concern for the sudden cutting of the ties with their beloved ones:

> I am influenced because we have no contacts at all and I have a hard time because of this. (Thanos, 36, Kastoria, employed, single)

> Relationship with my children is influenced because I have been isolated from them. We speak via internet, but we don't meet each other and I don't like this. The first week was fine but now I feel sad. (Mary, 68, Heraklion, retired, 2 kids)

In the same vein, Elena from Athens expresses high levels of dysthymia, worry and concern for this sudden restriction of physical contact:

> Relationship with my partner has become difficult: I live with my mother and I cannot meet him. He has to declare 'provision for vulnerable people' to be able to come to see me for an hour. This is a big problem for me as my relationship [with my partner] is sustained via Skype. [...]. I have been constrained a lot and this makes me feel dysthymia. Concerning familial

relationships, I live with my mother and I cannot even touch her; she works in a super market and this makes her vulnerable on the one hand and on the other hand, I should not get sick now [because of my pregnancy] so we have separated the house into two [...]. We had good news [pregnancy] and she did not hug me because we don't touch each other. (Elena, 35, Athens, employed, expecting)

The lack of contact has separated individuals from their intimates in a way that for many people is hardly manageable. The Covid-19 pandemic has affected the ways people interact with one another and had a tremendous impact on mental health (Cardenas et al., 2020). Intimate relationships are also affected especially for those partners who had not been living in the same country like in the cases of Lia from Brussels and Iason from Copenhagen:

My boyfriend lives in Greece and I cannot meet him. There is a climate of insecurity. (Lia, 28, Brussels, employed, single)

The problem is that my girlfriend is in England and I don't meet her. We are separated due to the circumstances. With parents we communicate via internet as before. I don't have the same personal contact with friends. (Iason 28, Copenhagen, unemployed, single)

As seen from the quotes above, lack of physical contact may generate feelings of sadness, uncertainly isolation and loneliness which in turn generate fear as already depicted by relevant literature (Zhou et al., 2020) and reflected in Theo's (from Northampton) fragment:

All the relationships have been influenced because there is no physical contact with anybody. Everything is done via telephone or SMS or nothing. Everyone's mind has turned into survival. And you are frightened. Since you are frightened, all relationships play second fiddle. [...]. Relationships will change and people will become cautious. (Theo, 41, Northampton, student, in relationship)

Notably, a different perspective views isolation as a familiar experience in everyday life as some older participants have depicted; for them, isolation and loneliness is not a new reality, and perhaps for that reason it may not be as difficult for them to cope with it. Dinos, Aristea and Nikos, all from Athens, reveal the same prolonged experience of isolation.

> No, I wouldn't say that relationships have been influenced. We speak on the phone with relatives even if we are all so depressive. With my child and grandchild we speak via internet. (Dinos, 84, Athens, retired, 1 kid)

> [Relationships did not change] Not at all. We are close with my husband as before. We communicate with friends via Skype as before. (Aristea, 65, Athens, housewife, married)

> Nothing changed. We speak with friends and we share our issues. And we anticipate for the best. (Nikos, 70, Athens, retired, married)

Loneliness and isolation seem to be part of normal way of living for some older people before and during the quarantine. Being used to social isolation as a result of a way of life can make social distancing less challenging and isolation less problematic (McKenna-Plumley et al., 2021). However, the quarantine has brought into light a lonely, isolated life showing the low quality of life for some individuals before the measures of social distancing.

In terms of theory, what has been explored can be integrated into the wider psychoanalytical framework of the relation with the object, meaning the process of developing a psyche in relation to others during childhood (Klein, 1952). Objects are usually internalised figures of mother, father or the primary caregiver. Internal objects (or the representations of the first caregivers) are created by the experiences of being taken care of as babies and the respective internalised images that one develops (Klein, 1930, 1932, 1952). Indeed, it is the particular accord our external world events with our earliest unconscious experiences on vulnerability and fright which makes these experiences so compelling. According to this theorisation, the participants of this section may feel unprotected and not taken care of. The "good mother" who can protect them does not exist (Klein, 1946); instead, what exists is the loss of "good mother" or the good life as we knew it until Covid-19. For some, this experience can constitute trauma. Isolation as perceived by Klein (1975) and restriction in physical contact influence relationships. Loss of established ways of living may be related to loss of the 'good mother', the security and familiarity of life before the implementation of lockdown measures.

Participants have discussed the impact of loss of contact through the emotions of discontent, sadness, worry concern and dysthymia. An additional aspect of isolation relates with separation of intimate relationship because of lockdown especially related to Greek diaspora, which involves feelings of sadness, uncertainty, and loneliness. As discussed in the previous chapters, fear is a distinct component of Covid-19 also depicted as experienced trauma. A rather distinctive perspective in relation to isolation derives from older participants, who express a familiarity with feelings of social isolation and loneliness due to their previous ways of life. The following section focuses on how the daily structures, routines and schedules have been modified as a result of the quarantine measures.

C. Disrupted Time Continuity

Disrupted rhythms of life in terms of time is one of the main consequences of the quarantine, also discussed in Chap. 5. One of the basic themes identified in participants' answers due to the disruption of their daily routines was the subsequent loss of the sense of time. Serious disruption of one's life continuity and of repetition of everyday experience by a sudden event or a sequence of events breaks the trust that one has in the continuity of life trajectory and the predictability of the world (Nicholson, 2010); existing defences against anxiety are overwhelmed and this can be traumatic. In this sense, and as discussed in the previous chapter, the rules of social isolation and quarantine can become a traumatic experience, where feelings of helplessness can generate fears of annihilation (Schejtman, 2021) and anxiety.

The examples below present this sudden disruption, entailing lack of interest in activities that participants loved before. Instead, there is a mood of boredom, loneliness and a sense that nothing changes. Theo from Northampton reflects this reality:

The day passes flatly: from the bed to the kitchen, to the toilet; internet and TV. [...]. The rhythms have decreased. My lessons have been transferred to online version. Anxiety has increased when I go out. [...]. Easter passed and there is no difference. Even TV programmes insert one in the mood that nothing changes. (Theo, 41, Northampton, student, in relationship)

Time passes and every day is the same; even religious celebrations, like Easter, so embedded into the Greek culture, are experienced as similar to any other day. In the same vein, Evi and Panos from Athens along with Kyriakos from Paris discuss intense daily transformations emphasising monotonous days, loss of time and purpose, lack of interest and boredom:

Of course [my daily routine] has changed. I used to be often outside of the house. I am rarely in home; just to eat and sleep [...]. Now it is the opposite, I have nothing to do outside [...]. My life is very monotonous but it passes quickly because my sleep is upside down and my partner's as well; we sleep very late and we wake up very late too. What happens is that we wake up, have coffee and lunch and we then navigate all the day on the laptop [...]. The day passes and we do nothing. We have no motivation to work for the University, for example. I become a procrastinator. (Evi, 21, Athens, in relationship, student)

Of course my everyday life has changed. I am very extrovert and this curfew has changed circumstances a lot. I go out only for super market or exercise around the house [...]. Due to this confinement time and days have been lost; sometimes, I lose the dates. [...]. I cannot get a rhythm and study for the University because it is difficult without having a deadline, a milestone to follow. So there is an invisible circle of decay in the house. A lot of videogames, YouTube, Netflix. A lot of time spent like that. (Panos, 21, Athens, student, in relationship)

I listen to music and I try to read books [...] but I don't read any more because of lack of interest or appetite. I do not exercise and I have been restrained in general. There are some websites where one can play videogames with play-station; however, I declare that I am bored. Boredom and lack of interest. (Kyriakos, 36, Paris, employed, single)

As participants explain, a lot of time is spent on screens and the internet, which can serve as a flight from the psychic pain caused due to the hard circumstances of the quarantine. Such examples can be seen as serious disruption of one's established defensive organisation. Individuals experience lack of interest in activities that they previously liked, monotony and boredom and loss of appetite and motivation to work; they are also faced with the time lost related to a sense of life with no purpose and meaning. Boredom indeed depends on a distorted sense of time in which time seems to stand still (Greenson, 1953, p. 7).

On the other hand, disruption of the routine and attempts towards a new structure of the day sometimes seem to co-exist and fight each other. There are individuals who seem to make an attempt to repair their sense of time and their daily rhythm by adding landmarks in their daily life such as physical activities and participating in outdoor activities that have turned online. Quarantine leads to the interruption of normal daily routine, working life and leisure activities; thus losing the days, and specific landmarks for each day may lead people to lose motivation (Dai & Li, 2019) whereas maintaining them seems to have helped several participants like Kostas and Zenia from Athens.

> My daily life has changed 40–50%. I used to work in the mornings which I do not do now. So, I sleep more in the mornings […] and I watch movies in the nights. So my rhythms have changed, I sleep later, I wake up later, I do the housework […] until my partner returns from work in the evenings […]. What has changed is that my time is differently structured. The evenings are the same but the mornings have changed a lot because I am alone in the house […]. I try to have activities during the day […]. And we have transferred our outdoor activities into online activities, such as our yoga lessons […]. We also use the screen more often than before. Up to now, we used the telephone for our needs but now it is a functional section of our lives. I can see my daughter only via the screen now. (Kostas, 60, Athens, employed, divorced, 2 kids)

> Yes, my daily life has changed a lot. Initially, we were used to sleep earlier so to wake up early and go to our job. But now we stay until late at night. One watches a lot of TV that s/he did not use to watch before. People can watch movies, serials […]. The positive thing is that we walk a lot; we did not walk so much in the past, we went to the gym. Now we have visited all the mountains of our area. We stay a lot in the house. Everything is different comparing to the past. (Zenia, 23, Athens, employed, single)

Time for oneself, studying or jogging are some activities that seemed to occupy individuals' time during the quarantine. There is more time available now for all, so people try to find new activities to keep them active. Furthermore, during quarantine, new activities have been adopted with an increase in time spent in front of a screen (Grondin et al., 2020). Characteristically, Aggeliki from Athens depicts the ways her daily routines have altered albeit in an adjustable manner:

> Everything is done with slower rhythms which I didn't have the opportunity to do before. I speak with friends via phone, I take my dog for a walk, I cook, I watch Netflix and I do not watch the news any more. It is creative because there is now time available that did not exist before. I have now the opportunity to do things for myself and for friends which is oxymoron. I feel happy that I don't need to go to work. I don't feel oppressed. (Aggeliki, 46, Athens, employed, in relationship, expecting)

Aggeliki explains the ways of filling up her days without feeling depressed by engaging in activities that keep her busy.

This section discussed the impact of the measure of social isolation during the April lockdowns in relation to disruption of time and life continuity. It was shown that such unsettlement has been experienced in a traumatic sense as social isolation measures generate boredom, which can affect the relationship individuals have with time, appearing slow, monotonous and long (Kumar & Nayar, 2020). Thus, loss of life before Covid-19 has been experienced as a disruption of time and life continuity either through monotony, boredom, loss of interest and purpose, or opportunity to reorganise everyday routines and restructure the ways time is spent. Once again, no regional specifications have been identified.

Participants' experience of Covid-19 as a traumatic event has been approached so far through core psychoanalytic understandings of the ways an experience of trauma can be analysed. Following relevant literature, Covid-19 has been analysed through experienced consequences of trauma in terms of (a) symbiosis, (b) isolation and (c) disruption of time continuity; these consequences have been identified regardless of the country of residence of the participants which indicates that shared experiences associated to the above-mentioned effects have not been limited to regional restrictions. Furthermore, an additional way that trauma can be approached is through collective trauma, as shared traumatic experiences ultimately lead to collective realities.

Collective Trauma of Loss

Collective trauma has been depicted as the collective response to a traumatising event which causes radical change and disruption within a short period of time (Neal, 1998) and is understood through the lived experiences of people who survived it (Erikson, 1976). Changes imposed because of the Covid-19 April 2020 lockdowns include social distancing, stay-at-home policies, travel restrictions, social isolation, and quarantines, increased vulnerabilities regarding mental health associated with post-traumatic symptoms (Brooks et al., 2020). Inevitably, such collective traumas may 'trigger' some people's un-remembered, suppressed past injuries (Okorn et al., 2020). Keeping in mind that collective trauma has been approached in different ways and is often associated with the impact on collective identities (Alexander, 2012), this section will concentrate on collective trauma solely in terms of collective loss of life prior to pandemic, as all participants have gone through this experience, while acknowledging that different people experience external devastating events in very different ways that depend on many different factors (Papadopoulos, 2007).

After discussing three broad consequences of Covid-19 as experienced trauma (symbiosis, isolation and disrupted time continuity), we shall now concentrate more directly on the loss of the life participants lived prior to the pandemic. Within this context, experienced collective trauma has been depicted according to the following two responses: (i) denial of the loss which generates persecutory anxieties and (ii) acceptance of the condition of loss through vulnerability and grief.

i) Denial of Loss

The first category includes fragments of participants who consciously or unconsciously, deny the loss that the pandemic entails. This category includes two subcategories of answers: (a) those who avoid/hide this loss with persecutory anxieties and (b) those who feel the omnipotence that people will be stronger after this pandemic.

Below there are some examples from the first subcategory, which concentrates on avoidance or denial of the loss of life prior to the pandemic through misbelief of the current reality; Michalis and Nikos from Athens discuss their beliefs about Covid-19 through suspicion and reluctance to accept reality:

I think that all this stilted. Of course, there is a virus which is contaminating. However, I think that the numbers (of deaths and cases) that are presented and the bad way they are presented, is a myth. How many people die of different diseases? They try to impose something else but I don't know what. They present the worst image rather than the reality. If they revealed the truth, nobody could stay at home and these measures and restrictions could not have passed for the reasons they desire. [...]. (Michalis, 48, Athens, employed, in relationship, expecting)

This is a challenge for all of us but I am sad because of the aim that all this happened. It is not an accident. (Nikos, 70, Athens, retired, married)

The quotes above implicate that there is a kind of conspiracy behind the pandemic, implying that some other people, identified as 'they', are trying to impose measures against the population for some suspicious reasons that are hidden from the public. Another perspective of this conspiracy comes from Aristea from Athens:

They want to break financially all the states. They want to reduce the population. They have achieved what they wanted; to reduce the population over 70 years old. I feel so bad for all this. (Aristea, 65, Athens, housewife, married)

In the quote above, the incentive is financial and the aim has been achieved. What is also implied is a splitting between "Them", the evil people who form conspiracies against "Us", the good and innocent victims of the global evil (Klein, 1946). The following quote by Dinos from Athens is covered by a religious veil, which bases its significance upon written religious records:

This is a serious challenge. The prophets have warned that famine and engulfment will come from Asia. I don't know if this is the truth or whether some people have constructed this as the truth. I think that it is suspicious that this happens all over the planet. In the past, diseases happened in specific areas. (Dinos, 84, Athens, retired, 1 kid)

What can be observed here is not the religious faith per se but the dogmatic attachment to religious ideas, which weaken an individual's intellectual ability, because it forecloses the possibilities of inquiry. What is common in all the above quotes is the sense of something hidden from the populations, a split between the good—pure people, the victims, the defeated, the devalued, the innocent—and the bad—evil, corrupted elite who exploit us, who desire to destroy and produce harm. The good qualities are projected upon "Us" the innocent people and the bad ones are projected upon the "bad others" (Klein, 1946). The depiction of such experienced reality may entail a primitive (or psychotic) mental functioning "making up the character of the paranoid-schizoid position and comprise denial, splitting, forms of projection and related identifications" (Hinshelwood, 1991). Thus, one way that denial of loss is reflected is through the avoidance of or suspicion towards the current reality.

The second subcategory consists of those who avoid or deny the loss of life prior to Covid-19 by viewing themselves and humanity as very strong and able to overcome it like Aggeliki from Athens and Aggelos from Los Angeles:

This crisis means a pause so we can see what happens inside us, outside of us and around us. And when the time comes for 'play again', one can check whether their life is as they desire, whether people around them are as they like, whether our job satisfies us. If something is not as we like it, we have to change it. This is a good chance for introspection because our life is so fast. Time passes and we don't have time to think. […] (Aggeliki, 46, Athens, employed, in relationship, expecting)

For me, [the pandemic] gave me a lot of time because after finishing my studies, I had the opportunity to prepare myself for interviews. So for me, the quarantine means a pause to time, a pause to my life; and it is upon us whether we will use this pause or just leave it untapped. Apart from that,

this is a very good experience: how to prepare and handle serious circumstances to show ourselves that we can handle it. Humans will always come
together for this better good. Everybody has acted well this situation especially in Greece. It is very pleasing that Greece has done so well. (Aggelos,
24, Los Angeles, employed part-time, single)

Aggeliki and Angelos could represent a positive view towards the pandemic because they speak about a pause as an opportunity for introspection and for life changes whereas at the same time they imply an avoidance
of the painful reality of the pandemic and its real circumstances for many
thousands of people; instead, they demonstrate an omnipotence that
humanity will respond efficiently to that and people will be stronger after
this. Of course, humanity may recover but one should also be capable of
acknowledging the difficult circumstances that many have been
experiencing.

Bill from Maryland reinforces the belief that people will be able to
overcome this pandemic:

We are all thrown down the river so to speak. We have to be aware of protecting our environment and ourselves. And if everybody does that then
there will be a better world to live in and healthier. (Bill, 78, Maryland,
retired, married)

What is implied here by Bill is that protecting the environment may
mean a deterrent factor for a pandemic or maybe that the lockdown
means less traffic and pollution. Whatever it means, the quote demonstrates that the humanity is strong enough to avoid the pandemic. Rita
from Germany views the pandemic as a natural phenomenon but with
no meaning and thus ultimately as an unimportant development:

Nothing. This crisis means absolutely nothing to me. It is a natural development. Pandemics always existed and will always exist; something happens every 50 years or so [...]. The bad news is that nowadays we feel
omnipotent. We feel that we have achieved everything and medicine has
reached its highest level. Ok, we are not so omnipotent but we are in a very
good level; I am satisfied with that. Imagine this pandemic with no means

of communication; this would be a problem and the lockdown would be awful, I assume. On the other hand, this is a natural flow; there is nothing shocking. […]. (Rita, 36, Germany, employed, single)

While Rita makes an accurate point, probably heard by scientific commentator in the media, it is the over-attention to this factor and complacent disregard for what it means in terms of heartache, premature loss and pain in others which is problematic. Both fragments reveal an avoidance or denial of reality and inability to acknowledge or accept the loss of life as it used to be, either through faith that this will also pass or through diminishing the significance of the pandemic.

This section depicts the aspect of denial as revealed in its various forms through participants' narratives. Denial was depicted through suspicion of a 'planned' pandemic, as the need to see the positive aspects of the pandemic, as a belief that this will pass or that this is the natural flow of the planet. The common element in this depiction of collective trauma relates to the way participants avoid or deny the acknowledgement or acceptance of loss of life as we knew it before the pandemic. Therefore, although shared trauma by a larger group is called 'collective trauma' in response to a mass traumatising event (Saul, 2013) (in this case lockdown measures), this does not mean that all people experience such event in the same manner. Indeed, this section depicted different ways of denying aspects or the whole of Covid-19 reality, although the experience has not affected these participants less than anyone else. Their response is marked by an omnipotence defence which blocks out the pain that would need to be felt in order to mourn the many kinds of loss the pandemic has enforced.

ii) Acceptance of Loss

A second category of narratives includes participants who seem to acknowledge the traumatic impact of the pandemic and accept the loss that it entails; this category includes narratives from participants a) who have adopted defences such as phobia or anxiety as well as narratives from participants (b) who may feel vulnerable and helpless while grieving the loss of their previous life. In both cases, the Covid-19 pandemic has been depicted as an event that has caused collective as well as personal trauma as it is activating traumatic memories of the historical past and turning it into destructive consequences for both individuals and groups (Kalsched, 2021). For example, Maria from Athens reveals her increased anxiety by stating:

> Nothing will be as before. The economic crisis that emerges is huge and I am afraid that we will face serious economic impacts. This makes me feel sadness, anxiety and uncertainty about the future. I never believed that an invisible enemy will influence so much life all over the planet. (Maria, 70, Athens, retired, 2 kids)

Maria is afraid about the future and especially the financial future, which makes people feel anxiety; such phobia is also depicted by Mary from Heraklion as she explains how circumstances have changed almost overnight, producing panic:

> When I went out and I realised that nobody comes out, I was scared. I said 'where am I?' I was in panic; we are nothing, overnight. Even if I am well at the moment but I feel so sad since I see what happens in other countries. […] We don't know how the next day will be. (Mary, 68, Crete, retired, 2 kids)

Feelings like the above, depict shared emotions of fear, anxiety and uncertainty of what will happen next. However, other participants emphasised shared feelings of vulnerability rather than panic and they seem to have adapted to the circumstances and have gone forward to mourning. Mourning is the reaction to the loss of the object, which here is normal life, security and a belief in the continuity of life, which no longer exists (Freud, 1926). The following fragments by Mari from Hong Kong, Thanos from Kastoria and Betty from Athens depict such shared reality:

> It is a crisis which we did not anticipate; it has changed our lives and we hope it will pass. But we don't know that. The most important for me is the inversion of everything we knew. Whatever planned is in the air and everything is unknown; circumstances are not so stable and especially for us who live abroad. (Mari, 40, Hong Kong, housewife, 1 kid)

How I feel? I laugh very often because I realise how small I am towards the nature [...]. And it's not about gloves and masks; it is just (the necessity) to master our fears. [...]. It is an accident if I am contaminated so let it be [...] I feel adrift and it is positive to think that we are all adrift. (Thanos, 36, Kastoria, employed, single)

It is an unpredictable evil which I am not prepared to face. [...] It will influence us all. We don't appreciate what we have and we don't prepare ourselves for the evil. This is a difficult situation which has not many things to offer apart from some opportunities and self-awareness thoughts. I wish people thought about that so we can make things better such as be more disciplined—as Greeks, we are not—or we can learn to have money or other goods in stock [...]. (Betty, 75, Athens, window, 2 kids)

The quotes above focus on the unpredictable character of the circumstances which have inverted people's certainties until recently. As discussed previously, many people were not prepared to face the disruption of the continuity of the daily routine and rhythms of life (Garland, 2002). The participants of this thematic category revealed acceptance of the loss of life as they knew it through reactions of (a) panic and anxiety as well as (b) vulnerability and mourning. One can see that the Covid-19 pandemic is shared not only nationally but also globally as it connects people around the world emotionally through experiences of helplessness, uncertainty, loss and grief (Watson et al., 2020).

This section discussed the different categories according to how the participants have experienced Covid-19 April 2020 lockdown as a collective trauma or loss of life prior to pandemic. Some of the features of the Covid-19 pandemic as a collective trauma include its sudden character that alters our normal life and rhythms, as the patterns of lives have been disrupted causing anxiety whereas the fear of death causes precariousness (Nikolo, 2021). Based on this depiction, fragments have been distinguished between those denying the traumatic loss of their previous life and those who have accepted the traumatic loss of their prior life through panic, anxiety and grief. Such mental states can be indicative of the mental states of people towards the trauma of the pandemic, the loss it entails and their responses towards it.

Synopsis

Rooted in psychoanalytic theory, this chapter explored experienced trauma through the loss of life as we knew it before Covid-19. Loss took several forms, including: (a) symbiosis, loss of space and time; (b) isolation, loss of physical and social contact as well as loss of quality of human contact; and (c) disrupted time continuity, loss through disruption of life and time continuity. Experienced trauma was also depicted collectively through (a) denial of loss as well as (b) acceptance of loss. This diversity of approaches to loss offered the opportunity to synthesise a rich plurality of shared experiences, shedding light on an experience of trauma through this pandemic.

Based on the participants' narratives, Covid-19 pandemic entailed the following distinct shared experiences:

a) Loss of space and time. Experienced trauma has been revealed in relation to closeness while living under the same roof with family members; experienced symbiosis revealed challenging aspects entailing fusion and merger (as well as fear towards these kinds of symbiosis), resulting in the loss of personal space and time imposed by continued cohabitation, a finding also revealed in relation to mothers. Additionally, primary symbiosis has also been disclosed as a form of mutual coverage of respective needs between family members. Closeness (and lack of) has been depicted through narratives deriving from the Greek diaspora emphasising the nostalgic need for contact with homeland and family.
b) Loss of established ways of living also includes isolation and restriction in physical contact, already identified in the previous chapter. Participants' narratives have reflected the impact of loss of contact through discontent, sadness, worry, concern and dysthymia. An additional aspect of isolation especially related to the Greek diaspora relates with separation of intimate relationship because of lockdown, which involves feelings of sadness, uncertainty, and loneliness. A rather distinctive perspective in relation to isolation derives from older participants, who express a familiarity with feelings of social isolation and loneliness due to their previous ways of life.

c) Loss of time and life continuity has been depicted through unsettlement (also analysed in Chap. 5 through transformations of everyday living and discontinuity of everyday life) which has been experienced in traumatic ways entailing loss of sense of time, purpose and interests for activities, boredom, loneliness and a sense that nothing changes. On the other hand, there are individuals who seem to make an attempt to repair their sense of time and their daily rhythm by adding landmarks in their daily life such as physical activities and participation in outdoor or online activities. Such activities have been depicted as opportunities for improvement. Thus, loss of life before Covid-19 has been experienced as disruption of time and life continuity either through monotony, boredom, loss of interest and purpose, or opportunity to reorganise everyday routines and restructure the ways time is spent and experienced.

d) Shared loss of life prior to the Covid-19 pandemic. This loss has been depicted through: (i) denial and (ii) acceptance of loss. The first category revealed avoidance or denial of the loss this pandemic entails including (a) those who avoid or hide this loss through suspicion and reluctance to accept reality and (b) those who feel the need to see the positive aspects of the pandemic, the belief that this will pass (also revealed through opportunities for improvement in the previous chapter) or that this is the natural flow of the planet. Both categories were in the form of omnipotent defences. The second thematic category revealed acceptance of the loss of life as they knew it through reactions of (a) panic and anxiety as well as (b) vulnerability and grief depicted previously through fearful conceptualisations of crisis.

Bibliography

Alexander, J. (2012). *Trauma: A Social Theory*. Polity.

Angel, K. (1967). On Symbiosis and Pseudosymbiosis. *Journal of American Psychoanalytic Association, 15*, 294–315.

Angel, K. (1972). The Role of the Internal Object and External Object in Object-Relationships, Separation Anxiety, Object Constancy and Symbiosis. *International Journal of Psychoanalysis, 53*, 541–546.

Blass, R. B., & Blatt, S. J. (1996). Attachment and Separateness in the Experience of Symbiotic Relatedness. *The Psychoanalytic Quarterly, 65*(4), 711–746. https://doi.org/10.1080/21674086.1996.11927513

Brooks, S. K., Webster, R. K., Smith, L. E., Woodland, L., Wessely, S., Greenberg, N., & Rubin, G. J. (2020). The Psychological Impact of Quarantine and How to Reduce it: Rapid Review of the Evidence. *Lancet, 395*(10227), 912–920.

Cardenas, M. C., Bustos, S. S., & Chakraborty, R. (2020). A 'parallel pandemic': The Psychosocial Burden of COVID-19 in Children and Adolescents. *Acta pædiatrica, 109*(11), 2187–2188.

Dai, H., & Li, C. (2019). How Experiencing and Anticipating Temporal Landmarks Influence Motivation. *Current Opinion in Psychology, 26*, 44–48. https://doi.org/10.1016/j.copsyc.2018.04.012

Erikson, K. (1976). *Everything in its Path: Destruction on Community in the Buffalo Creek Flood.* Simon and Schuster.

Freud, A. (1936). *The Ego and the Mechanisms of Defense.* International Universities Press.

Freud, S. (1917). Introductory Lectures on Psycho-Analysis. *The Standard Edition of the Complete Psychological Works of Sigmund Freud*, Volume XVI (1916–1917): Introductory Lectures on Psycho-Analysis (Part III), 241–463.

Freud, S. (1920). Beyond the Pleasure Principle. *The Standard Edition of the Complete Psychological Works of Sigmund Freud, 18*, 1–64.

Freud, S. (1926). Inhibitions, Symptoms and Anxiety. *The Standard Edition of the Complete Psychological Works of Sigmund Freud, 20*, 75–176.

Garland, C. (2002). *Understanding Trauma: A Psychoanalytical Approach.* Karnac Books. Second Enlarged Edition. First Published in 1998

Greenson, R. R. (1953) On Boredom. *Journal of the American Psychoanalytic Association, 1*, 7–21 (p. 20)

Grondin, S., Mendoza-Duran, E., & Rioux, P. A. (2020). Pandemic, Quarantine, and Psychological Time. *Frontiers in psychology, 11*, 581036. https://doi.org/10.3389/fpsyg.2020.581036

Harrison, I. B. (1986). On "merging" and the Phantasy of Merging. *Psychoanalytic Study of the Child, 41*, 155–170.

Hinshelwood, R. D. (1991). *A Dictionary of Kleinian thought.* Free Association Books.

Jiao, W. Y., Wang, L. N., Liu, J., Fang, S. F., Jiao, F. Y., Pettoello-Mantovani, M., & Somekh, E. (2020). Behavioral and Emotional Disorders in Children during the COVID-19 Epidemic. *The Journal of Pediatrics., 17*(3), 230–233.

Kalsched, D. (2021). Intersections of Personal vs. Collective Trauma during the COVID-19 Pandemic: The Hijacking of the Human Imagination. *Journal of Analytical Psychology, 66*(3), 443–462.

Klein, M. (1930). The Importance of Symbol-Formation in the Development of the Ego. *International Journal of Psychoanalysis, 11*, 24–39.

Klein, M. (1932). X. The Significance of Early Anxiety-Situations in the Development of the Ego. *The Psycho-Analysis of Children, 22*, 245–267.

Klein, M. (1935). A Contribution to the Psychogenesis of Manic-Depressive States. *International Journal of Psychoanalysis, 16*, 145–174.

Klein, M. (1946). Notes on Some Schizoid Mechanisms. *International Journal of Psychoanalysis, 27*, 99–110.

Klein, M. (1952). The Origins of Transference. *International Journal of Psychoanalysis, 33*, 433–438.

Klein, M. (1955). On Identification. In *Envy and Gratitude: A study of Unconscious Sources* (pp. 141–175). Delacorte Press.

Klein, M. (1975). Envy and Gratitude and Other Works 1946–1963: Edited By: M. Masud R. Khan. *Envy and Gratitude and Other Works* 1946–1963 104:1–346.

Kumar, A., & Nayar, K. R. (2020). COVID 19 and its Mental Health Consequences. *Journal of Mental Health, 27*, 1–2. https://doi.org/10.108 0/09638237.2020.1757052

Laplanche, J., & Pontalis, J. B. (1981). *Leksilogio tis psichanalisis [The Dictionary of Psychoanalysis]*. Kedros Publications.

Mahler, M. S., Pine, F., & Bergman, A. (1975). *The Psychological Birth of the Human Infant: Symbiosis and Individuation*. Basic Books.

McKenna-Plumley, P. E., Graham-Wisener, L., Berry, E., & Groarke, J. M. (2021). Connection, Constraint, and Coping: A Qualitative Study of Experiences of Loneliness during the COVID-19 Lockdown in the UK. *PLoS ONE, 16*(10), e0258344. https://doi.org/10.1371/journal.pone.0258344

Meissner, W. W. (1981). Metapsychology—Who Needs It? *Journal of American Psychoanalytic Association, 29*, 921–938.

Nacht, S. (1964). Silence as an Integrative Factor. *International Journal of Psychoanalysis., 45*, 299–303.

Neal, A. G. (1998). *National Trauma and Collective Memory: Major Events in the American Century*. M. E. Sharpe, Armonk.

Nicholson, C. (2010). *Children and Adolescents in Trauma. Creative Therapeutic Approaches* (C. Nicholson, M. Irwin, & K. N. Dwivendi, Eds.). Jessica Kingsley Publishers.

Nikolo, A. M. (2021). The COVID 19 Pandemic and Individual and Collective Trauma. *International Journal of Applied Psychoanalytic Studies, 1*, 1–6.

Okorn, I., et al. (2020). Isolation in the COVID-19 Pandemic as Re-traumatization of War Experiences. *Croat Med Journal, 61*, 371–376.

Papadopoulos, R. (2007). Refugees, Trauma and Adversity-Activated Development. *European Journal of Psychotherapy and Counselling, 9*(3), 301–312. https://doi.org/10.1080/13642530701496930

Pollock, G. (1964). On Symbiosis and Symbiotic Neurosis. *International Journal of Psychoanalysis, 45*, 1–30.

Rose, G. J. (1964). Creative Imagination in Terms of Ego 'core' and boundaries. *International Journal of Psychoanalysis., 45*, 75–84.

Rose, G. J. (1972). Fusion States. In P. L. Giovaccini (Ed.), *Tactics and Techniques in Psychoanalytic Psychotherapy* (pp. 170–188). Science House.

Saul, J. (2013). *Collective Trauma, Collective Healing: Promoting Community Resilience in the Aftermath of Disaster* (Vol. 48). Routledge.

Schejtman, C. R. (2021). Coping with Pandemic, Psychoanalytical Interventions with Parents and Children: Institutional and Community Approaches. *International Journal of Applied Psychoanalytic Studies, 18*(2), 177–187.

Watson, M. F., Bacigalupe, G., Daneshpour, M., Han, W. J., & Parra-Cardona, R. (2020). COVID-19 Interconnectedness: Health Inequity, the Climate Crisis, and Collective Trauma. *Family Process., 59*(2), 832–843.

Zhou, S.-J., Zhang, L.-G., Wang, L.-L., et al. (2020). Prevalence and Socio-demographic Correlates of Psychological Health Problems in Chinese Adolescents during the Outbreak of COVID-19. *European Child & Adolescent Psychiatry, 29*, 749–758.

Correction to: Psycho-Social Approaches to the Covid-19 Pandemic

Correction to:

A. Chalari, E. E. Koutantou, *Psycho-Social Approaches to the Covid-19 Pandemic*, https://doi.org/10.1007/978-3-031-07831-6

The book was inadvertently published with an incorrect spelling of the author's name as Anathasia Chalari. The correct name Athanasia Chalari has been updated.

The updated original version for this book can be found at
https://doi.org/10.1007/978-3-031-07831-6

Epilogue

Having completed this journey through participants' experiences, it is time to offer the answer to the core question of this book: What does this pandemic mean? The meaning-making of this pandemic entailed a plurality of emotions associated with the impact of the pandemic on different aspects of life primarily associated with change, crisis and trauma. Inevitably, the answer to this question entails a shorter and a longer response.

The former concentrates on the affected areas of life and can be summarised as follows:

The Covid-19 pandemic has been portrayed as a radical economic, political and social change, as well as a transformation of everyday life; it has been experienced as unsettlement and disruption of life continuity and has been narrated as a fearful crisis also entailing opportunity for improvement. The traumatic aspect of the pandemic has been encountered as loss of space and time, loss of established ways of living, loss of time and life continuity as well as denial or acceptance of the loss of life prior to Covid-19.

A. Chalari, E. E. Koutantou, *Psycho-Social Approaches to the Covid-19 Pandemic*, https://doi.org/10.1007/978-3-031-07831-6

The latter concentrates on the depiction of emotions which requires a more detailed response:

The pandemic has been depicted as (a) *radical economic, political and social changes* that caused fear, uncertainty, anger abandonment and tension as well as (b) *a transformation of everyday life* causing disappointment, anger, distrust and uncertainty affecting particularly parents (predominantly mothers), due to the devotion of their personal time/space to work, family and online schooling. It has been perceived as *unsettlement and disruption* of life continuity entailing feelings of being: surprised, cornered, depressed, imprisoned and even immobilised because of uncertainty, including feelings of an incomplete life, a life not lived, characterised by dead time.

The pandemic has also been portrayed as (a) a fearful *crisis*: entailing panic, sadness, vulnerability, uncertainty and a failure of humanity as well as (b) an opportunity for improvement through self and social awareness and evaluation, optimism, hopefulness, patience, empathy, caring, understanding, respect, love, humour, gratitude and self-support. Ultimately, portraying crisis as an opportunity rather than as fear enabled participants to concentrate on the means employed to cope with the pandemic.

The traumatic aspects of this pandemic have also been illustrated through: *loss of space and time* which resulted to symbiosis and cohabitation. The Greek diaspora was particularly affected through loss of closeness to homeland; *loss of established ways of living* including isolation, and the restriction in physical contact caused discontent, sadness, worry, concern and dysthymia. Separation from intimate relationships affected particularly Greek diaspora causing feelings of sadness, uncertainty, isolation and loneliness whereas older participants have expressed familiarity with feelings of social isolation and loneliness; *loss of time and life continuity* caused feelings of loss of sense of time, of purpose and interests for activities, boredom, loneliness and a sense that nothing changes. However, some have made attempts to repair their sense of time and their daily rhythm by adding landmarks in their daily life such as physical activities and participation in outdoor or online activities.

Finally, the pandemic has been narrated through *shared loss of life prior* to the Covid-19 pandemic and resulted in (i) *denial of the loss* this pandemic entails by (a) those who avoid or hide this loss through suspicion and reluctance to accept reality and (b) those who feel the need to see only the positive aspects of the pandemic, the belief that this will pass or that this is the natural flow of the planet; (ii) *acceptance of the loss* of life prior to Covid-19 through reactions of (a) panic and anxiety as well as (b) vulnerability and grief.

Overall, it seems justified to argue that, lived experiences of Covid-19 pandemic among the participants of this study have not been differentiated according to regional specifications. Furthermore, the analysis of this data did not detect profound patterns among participants associated with class, educational or employment specifications. Distinctive patterns were depicted in relation to social isolation among mothers, in terms of shared experiences of loss of time and space; among older participants, regarding familiarity with feelings of isolation and loneliness and Greek diaspora, in relation to feelings of nostalgia, separation and abandonment. In broader terms, the analysed fragments of the participants allowed a synthesis of the meaning-making of the Covid-19 pandemic through their lived experiences, regardless of their regional residence at the time of the April 2020 lockdown.

Reaching the completion of this endeavour, we come to realise that the ways this pandemic has been portrayed so far remain incomplete. Although the study of the pandemic's aftermath has and will remain an infinite source of exploration, we need to remember that, after all, the ultimate source of understanding the meaning of such a complex reality can only derive from first-hand experiences occurring in real time. And as the exploration of human experience might only be compared to the expansive exploration of the universe, any attempt to do so inevitably creates even more questions than the ones answered. Luckily, this is the purpose of synergies between different disciplines like the one attempted in this book, between sociological and psychosocial approaches. In facing a global pandemic which does not respond to boundaries and barriers, it seems all the more important to join forces in order to offer deeper and more complete understandings of how human experiences may transform into meaning-making, albeit also opening up new windows to unexplored aspects of social and personal realities.

Bibliography

Abramson, L. Y., Metalsky, G. I., & Alloy, L. B. (1989). Hopelessness Depression: A Theory-based Subtype of Depression. *Psychological Review., 96*, 358–372. https://doi.org/10.1037/0033-295X.96.2.358

Alexander, J. (2012). *Trauma: a Social Theory.* Polity.

Alvesson, M. (2002). *Postmodernism and Social Research.* Open University Press.

Angel, K. (1967). On Symbiosis and Pseudosymbiosis. *Journal of American Psychoanalytic Association, 15*, 294–315.

Angel, K. (1972). The Role of the Internal Object and External Object in Object-Relationships, Separation Anxiety, Object Constancy and Symbiosis. *International Journal of Psychoanalysis, 53*, 541–546.

Anwar, A., Malik, M., & Raees, V. (2020). Role of Mass Media and Public Health Communications in the COVID-19 Pandemic. *Cureus, 12*, e10453–e10453.

Asmundson, G. J. G., & Taylor, S. (2020). Coronaphobia: Fear of the 2019-nCoV Outbreak. *Journal of Anxiety Disorders, 70*, 102196.

Bacevic, J., & McGoey, L. (2021). *Surfing Ignorance: Covid-19 and the Rise of Fatalistic Liberalism, Research Repository.* University of Essex (Unpublished). http://repository.essex.ac.uk/30721/

Baker, C. (1997). Membership Categorisation and Interview Accounts. In D. Silverman (Ed.), *Qualitative Research.* Sage.

Bao, Y., Sun, Y., Meng, S., Shi, J., & Lu, L. (2020). 2019-nCoV Epidemic: Address Mental Health Care to Empower Society. *Lancet, 395*(10224), e37–e38.

Bartley, M. (2006). *Capability and Resilience: Beating the Odds*. University College London, Department of Epidemiology and Public Health.

Battyany, K. (2020). The Covid-19 Pandemic Reveals and Exacerbates the Crisis of Care. *Open Democracy*. https://www.opendemocracy.net/en/openmovements/covid-19-pandemic-reveals-and-exacerbates-crisis-care/

Becker, H., & S. (1963). *Outsiders: Studies in the Sociology of Deviance*. Free Press.

Benke, C., Autenrieth, L. K., Asselmann, E., & Pané-Farré, C. A. (2020). Lockdown, Quarantine Measures, and Social Distancing: Associations with Depression, Anxiety and Distress at the Beginning of the COVID-19 Pandemic Among Adults from Germany. *Psychiatry Research, 293*, 113462.

Best, L. A., Law, M. A., Roach, S., & Wilbiks, J. M. P. (2020). The Psychological Impact of COVID-19 in Canada: Effects of Social Isolation During the Initial Response. *Canadian Psychology*. https://doi.org/10.1037/cap0000254

Blass, R. B., & Blatt, S. J. (1996). Attachment and Separateness in the Experience of Symbiotic Relatedness. *The Psychoanalytic Quarterly, 65*(4), 711–746. https://doi.org/10.1080/21674086.1996.11927513

Bohleber, W. (2010). *Destructiveness, Intersubjectivity and Trauma*. Routledge.

Bohlken, J., Schömig, F., Lemke, M. R., Pumberger, M., & Riedel-Heller, S. G. (2020). COVID-19 pandemic: Stress Experience of Healthcare Workers: A Short Current Review. *Psychiatrische Praxis, 47*, 190–197.

Boniol, M., McIsaac, M., Xu, L., Wuliji, T., Diallo, K., & Campbell, J. (2019). *Gender Equity in the Health Workforce: Analysis of 104 Countries*. World Health Organization. https://apps.who.int/iris/bitstream/handle/10665/311314/WHOHIS-HWF-Gender-WP1-2019.1-eng.pdf

Bonsaksen, T., Heir, T., Schou-Bredal, I., Ekeberg, Ø., Skogstad, L., & Grimholt, T. K. (2020). Post-traumatic Stress Disorder and Associated Factors during the Early Stage of the COVID-19 Pandemic in Norway. *International Journal of Environmental Research and Public Health, 17*, 9210. https://doi.org/10.3390/ijerph17249210

Brooks, S. K., Webster, R. K., Smith, L. E., Woodland, L., Wessely, S., Greenberg, N., & Rubin, G. J. (2020). The Psychological Impact of Quarantine and How to Reduce it: Rapid review of the Evidence. *Lancet, 395*(10227), 912–920.

Brown, R. D. (2020). Public Health Lessons Learned from Biases in Coronavirus Mortality Overestimation. *Disaster Medicine and Public Health Preparedness, 14*, 1–24.

BSA. (2022). *Guidelines on Ethical Research*. British Sociological Association. https://www.britsoc.co.uk/ethics

Caduff, C. (2020). What Went Wrong: Corona and the World After the Full Stop. *Medical Anthropology Quarterly, 34*(4), 467–487.

Calhoun, C. (1992). Social Change. In E. F. Borgatta & M. L. Borgatta (Eds.), *Encyclopedia of Sociology* (Vol. 4, pp. 1807–1812). Macmillan.

Calnan, M. (2020). Health Policy and Controlling Covid-19 in England: Sociological Insights. *Emerald Open Research, 2*(40), 2–14. https://doi.org/10.35241/emeraldopenres.13726.2

Cardenas, M. C., Bustos, S. S., & Chakraborty, R. (2020). A 'parallel pandemic': The Psychosocial Burden of COVID-19 in Children and Adolescents. *Acta pædiatrica, 109*(11), 2187–2188.

Caruth, C. (1995). Unclaimed Experience: Trauma Narrative and History. In C. Caruth (Ed.), *Trauma: Explorations in Memory*. John Hopkins University Press.

Cauberghe, V., De Jans, S., Hudders, L., & Vanwesenbeeck, I. (2021). Children's Resilience during Covid-19 Confinement. A Child's Perspective–Which General and Media Coping Strategies are Useful? *Journal of Community Psychology, 50*, 1–18.

Cellini, N., Canale, N., Mioni, G., & Costa, S. (2020). Changes in Sleep Pattern, Sense of Time and Digital Media Use during COVID-19 Lockdown in Italy. *Journal of Sleep Res., 29*, e13074. https://doi.org/10.1111/jsr.13074

Chao, M., Chen, X., Liu, T., Yang, H., & Hall, B. J. (2020). Psychological Distress and State Boredom during the Covid 19 Outbreak in China: The Role of Meaning in Life and Media Use in European. *Journal of Psychot raumatology, 11*(1), 1769379.

Charmaz, K., & Belgrave, L. L. (2015). Grounded Theory. In G. Ritzer (Ed.), *The Blackwell Encyclopedia of Sociology*. John Wiley & Sons.

Collins, C., Landivar, L. C., Ruppanner, L., & Scarborough, W. J. (2020). COVID-19 and the Gender Gap in Work Hours. *Gender, Work & Organization*. https://doi.org/10.1111/gwao.12506.

Cooke, J. E., Eirich, R., Racine, N., & Madigan, S. (2020). Prevalence of Posttraumatic and General Psychological Stress during COVID-19: A Rapid Review and Meta-analysis. *Psychiatry Research., 292*, 113347. https://doi.org/10.1016/j.psychres.2020.113347

Dai, H., & Li, C. (2019). How Experiencing and Anticipating Temporal Landmarks Influence Motivation. *Current Opinion in Psychology., 26*, 44–48. https://doi.org/10.1016/j.copsyc.2018.04.012

David, C. (1980). Metapsychological Reflections on the Stage of Being in Love. In S. Lebovici & D. Widlocher (Eds.), *Psychoanalysis in France* (pp. 87–109). International University Press.

Demertzis, N., & Eyerman, R. (2020). Covid-19 as Cultural Trauma. *American Journal of Cultural Sociology, 8*, 428–450. https://doi.org/10.1057/s41290-020-00112-z

Dinerstein, A. C., Schwartz, G., & Taylor, G. (2014). Sociological Imagination as Social Critique: Interrogating the 'Global Economic Crisis. *Sociology, 48*(5), 859–868.

Droit-Volet, S., Gil, S., Martinelli, N., Andant, N., Clinchamps, M., Parreira, L., et al. (2020). Time and Covid-19 stress in the Lockdown Situation: Time free, «Dying» of Boredom and Sadness. *PLoS One, 15*, e0236465. https://doi.org/10.1371/journal.pone.0236465

Du, J., Dong, L., Wang, T., Yuan, C., Rao, F., Zhang, L., Liu, B., Zhang, M., Yin, Y., Qin, J., Bouey, J., Zhao, M., & Li, X. (2020). Psychological Symptoms among Frontline Healthcare Workers during COVID-19 Outbreak in Wuhan. *General Hospital Psychiatry, 67*, 144–145.

Duan, L., & Zhu, G. (2020). Psychological Interventions for People Affected by the COVID-19 Epidemic. *Lancet Psychiatry, 7*(4), 300–302.

Durkheim, E. (1933[1893]). *The Division of Labor in Society* (G. Simpson, Trans.). The Free Press.

Durkheim, E. (1951[1897]). *Suicide: A Study in Sociology* (J. A. Spaulding & G. Simpson, Trans.). The Free Press.

Elder, G. H. (1974/1999). *Children of the Great Depression: Social Change in Life Experience*. Westview Press. [First published 1974].

Elder, G. H., Jr., & Caspi, A. (1990). Studying Lives in a Changing Society: Sociological and Personological Explorations. In A. I. Rabin, R. A. Zucker, R. A. Emmons, & S. Frank (Eds.), *Studying Persons and Lives* (pp. 201–247). Springer Publishing Co.

Erikson, K. (1976). *Everything in its Path: Destruction on Community in the Buffalo Creek Flood*. Simon and Schuster.

Esterberg, K. G. (2002). *Qualitative Methods in Social Research*. McGraw Hill.

Frankl, V. (1959). *Man's Search for Meaning*. Washington Square Press.

French, S., Leyshon, A., & Thrift, N. (2009). A Very Geographical Crisis: The Making and Breaking of the 2007–2008 Financial Crisis. *Cambridge Journal of Regions, Economy and Society, 2*(2), 287–302.

Freud, A. (1936). *The Ego and the Mechanisms of Defense*. International Universities Press.

Freud, S. (1893). Charcot. *The Standard Edition of the Complete Psychological Works of Sigmund Freud, 3*, 7–23.

Freud, S. (1896). The Aetiology of Hysteria. *The Standard Edition of the Complete Psychological Works of Sigmund Freud, 3*, 191–221.

Freud, S. (1917). Introductory Lectures on Psycho-Analysis. *The Standard Edition of the Complete Psychological Works of Sigmund Freud*, Volume XVI (1916–1917): Introductory Lectures on Psycho-Analysis (Part III), 241–463.

Freud, S. (1920). *Beyond the Pleasure Principle SE.*

Freud, S. (1926). Inhibitions, Symptoms and Anxiety. *The Standard Edition of the Complete Psychological Works of Sigmund Freud, 20*, 75–176.

Frosh, S. (2010). *Psychoanalysis Outside the Clinic. Interventions in Psychosocial Studies.* Palgrave Macmillan.

Frosh, S., & Emerson, P. (2004). Interpretation and Over-interpretation: Disrupting the Meaning of Texts. *Qualitative Research, 5*(3), 307–324.

Frosh, S., Phoenix, A., & Pattman, R. (2003). Taking a Stand: Using Psychoanalysis to Explore the Positioning of Subjects in Discourse. *British Journal of Social Psychology, 42*(1), 39–53. https://doi. org/10.1348/014466603763276117

Frosh, S., & Saville, Y. (2011). Psychoanalytic Approaches to Qualitative Psychology. In C. Willig & W. Stainton-Rogers (Eds.), *The SAGE Handbook of Qualitative Research in Psychology* (pp. 109–126). SAGE.

Fuchs, C. (2020). 'Everyday Life and Everyday Communication in Coronavirus Capitalism', Triple C: Communication, Capitalism & Critique. *Open Access Journal for a Global Sustainable Information Society, 18*(1), 375–398.

Gadamer, H.-G. (1976). *Philosophical Hermeneutics.* University of California Press.

Gadamer, H.-G. (2004). *Truth and Method.* Continuum Publishing Group.

Garland, C. (2002). *Understanding Trauma: A Psychoanalytical Approach.* Karnac Books. Second Enlarged Edition. First published in 1998

Goh, K. K., Lu, M. L., & Jou, S. (2020). 'Impact of COVID-19 Pandemic: Social Distancing and the Vulnerability to Domestic Violence. *Psychiatry and Clinical Neurosciences', 74*(11), 612–613.

Gordon, A. (2008). *Ghostly Matters Haunting and the Sociological Imagination.* University of Minnesota Press.

Gori, A., & Topino, E. (2021). Across the COVID-19 Waves—Assessing Temporal Fluctuations in Perceived Stress, Post-traumatic Symptoms, Worry, Anxiety and Civic Moral Disengagement Over One Year of Pandemic. *International Journal of Environmental Research and Public Health, 18*(11), 5651.

Grasso, M., Klicperová-Baker, M., Koos, S., Kosyakova, Y., Petrillo, A., & Vlase, I. (2020). The Impact of the Coronavirus Crisis on European Societies., What Have We Learned and Where Do We Go from Here? Introduction to the Covid Volume. *European Societies., 23*(S1), 2–32.

Grondin, S., Mendoza-Duran, E., & Rioux, P. A. (2020). Pandemic, Quarantine, and Psychological Time. *Frontiers in psychology, 11*, 581036. https://doi.org/10.3389/fpsyg.2020.581036

Grunberger, B. (1971). *Narcissism: Psychoanalytic Essays.* International University Press. 1979.

Guo, J., Feng, X. L., Wang, X. H., & van I Jzendoorn, M. H. C. (2020). Coping with COVID-19: Exposure to COVID-19 and Negative Impact on Livelihood Predict Elevated Mental Health Problems in Chinese Adults. *International Journal of Environmental Research and Public Health, 17*, 3857.

Hall, S. M. (2019). A Very Personal Crisis: Family Fragilities and Everyday Conjunctures Within Lived Experiences of Austerity. *Transactions of the Institute of British Geographers, 44*, 479–492.

Harris, D., Ellis, D. Y., Gorman, D., Foo, N., & Haustead, D. (2021). Impact of COVID-19 Social Restrictions on Trauma Presentations in South Australia. *Emergency Medicine Australasia, 33*(1), 152–154.

Harrison, I. B. (1986). On "merging" and the Phantasy of Merging. *Psychoanalytic Study of the Child, 41*, 155–170.

Hellinism.net. (2022). Retrieved June 15, 2022, from https://hellenism.net/greece/greek-culture/greek-diaspora/

Hirschberger, G. (2018). Collective Trauma and the Social Construction of Meaning. *Frontiers in Psychology, 9*, 1–14.

Hoaglin, D., Mosteller, F., & Tukey, J. W. (1983). *Understanding Robust and Exploratory Data Analysis.* Wiley.

Hollway, W., & Jefferson, T. (2000). *Doing Qualitative Research Differently: Free Association Narrative and the Interview Method.* SAGE.

Home. (2020, July). Collective Trauma Amid Covid: Excerpt from 'Together Apart'. https://www.socialsciencespace.com/2020/07/collective-trauma-amid-covid-excerpt-from-together-apart/

Jacobson, E. (1964). *The Self and the Object World.* International University Press.

Jiao, W. Y., Wang, L. N., Liu, J., Fang, S. F., Jiao, F. Y., Pettoello-Mantovani, M., & Somekh, E. (2020). Behavioral and Emotional Disorders in Children during the COVID-19 Epidemic. *The Journal of Pediatrics, 17*(3), 230–233.

Jowett, A. (2021). Currying out Qualitative Research under Lockdown -Practical and Ethical Considerations. *LSE Impact Block.* https://blogs.lse.ac.uk/impactofsocialsciences/2020/04/20/carrying-out-qualitative-research-under-lockdown-practical-and-ethical-considerations/

Kalsched, D. (2021). Intersections of Personal vs. Collective Trauma during the COVID-19 Pandemic: The Hijacking of the Human Imagination. *Journal of Analytical Psychology, 66*(3), 443–462.

Kearns, M., Muldoon, O. T., Msetfi, R. M., & Surgenor, P. W. G. (2017). Darkness into Light? Identification with the Crowd at a Suicide Prevention Fundraiser Promotes Well-being Amongst Participants. *European Journal of Social Psychology, 47*(7). https://doi.org/10.1002/ejsp.2304

Klein, M. (1930). The Importance of Symbol-Formation in the Development of the Ego. *International Journal of Psychoanalysis, 11*, 24–39.

Klein, M. (1932). X. The Significance of Early Anxiety-Situations in the Development of the Ego. *The Psycho-Analysis of Children, 22*, 245–267.

Klein, M. (1935). A Contribution to the Psychogenesis of Manic-Depressive States. *International Journal of Psychoanalysis, 16*, 145–174.

Klein, M. (1946). Notes on Some Schizoid Mechanisms. *International Journal of Psychoanalysis, 27*, 99–110.

Klein, M. (1952). The Origins of Transference. *International Journal of Psychoanalysis, 33*, 433–438.

Klein, M. (1955). On Identification. In *Envy and Gratitude: A study of Unconscious Sources* (pp. 141–175). Delacorte Press.

Klein, M. (1975). Envy and Gratitude and Other Works 1946–1963: Edited By: M. Masud R. Khan. *Envy and Gratitude and Other Works 1946–1963* 104:1–346.

Koselleck, R., & Richter, M. W. (2006). Crisis. *Journal of the History of Ideas, 67*(2), 357–400.

Kumar, A., & Nayar, K. R. (2020). COVID 19 and its Mental Health Consequences. *Journal of Mental Health, 27*, 1–2. https://doi.org/10.108 0/09638237.2020.1757052

Kvale, S. (1996). *Inter Views: An Introduction to Qualitative Research Interviewing.* Sage.

Laplanche, J., & Pontalis, J. B. (1973). The Language of Psycho-Analysis: Translated by Donald Nicholson-Smith. *The Language of Psycho-Analysis, 94*, 1–497.

Laplanche, J., & Pontalis, J. B. (1981). *Leksilogio tis psichanalisis [The Dictionary of Psychoanalysis].* Kedros Publications.

Lazarus R. S., & Folkman S. (1984). Stress, Appraisal and Coping. New York: Springer.

Lewin, K. (1942). Time Perspective and Morale. In G. Watson (Ed.), *Civilian Morale* (pp. 48–70). Houghton Mifflin.

Lewis, A. B., Jr., & Landis, B. (1973). Symbiotic Pairings in Adults. *Contemporary Psychoanalysis, 9*(2), 230–249. https://doi.org/10.1080/00107530.1973.10745277

Light, R. J., Singer, J., & Willet, J. (1990). *By Design: Conducting Research on Higher Education*. Harvard University Press.

Lindinger-Sternart, S., Kaur, V., Widyaningsih, Y., & Patel, A. K. (2021). COVID-19 Phobia Across the World: Impact of Resilience on COVID-19 Phobia in Different Nations. *Counselling and Psychotherapy Research, 21*(2), 290–302.

Lourens, M. (2020, April 19). A Snapshot of Lockdown Shows Big Changes. *Sunday Star-Times*, 2–3.

Mahler, M. S., Pine, F., & Bergman, A. (1975). *The Psychological Birth of the Human Infant: Symbiosis and Individuation*. Basic Books.

Marasinghe, K. M. (2020). Face Mask Use Among Individuals Who Are Not Medically Diagnosed with COVID-19: A Lack of Evidence for and Against and Implications around Early Public Health Recommendations. *International Journal of One Health, 6*(2), 109–117. https://doi.org/10.14202/IJOH.2020.109-117

Masten, A. S. (2001). Ordinary Magic: Resilience Processes in Development. *American Psychologist, 56*(3), 227–238.

Matthewman, S., & Huppatz, K. (2020). A Sociology of Covid-19. *Journal of Sociology, 46*(4), 675–683.

Maxwell, J. A. (2013). *Qualitative Research Design: an Interactive Approach*. Sage.

May, V. (2011). Self, Belonging and Social Change. *Sociology, 45*(3), 363–378.

McKenna-Plumley, P. E., Graham-Wisener, L., Berry, E., & Groarke, J. M. (2021). Connection, Constraint, and Coping: A Qualitative Study of Experiences of Loneliness during the COVID-19 lockdown in the UK. *PLoS ONE, 16*(10), e0258344. https://doi.org/10.1371/journal.pone.0258344

Meerloo, J. (1962). The Dual Meaning of Human Regression. *Psychoanalytic Review, (49) (3)*, 77–86.

Meissner, W. W. (1981). Metapsychology—Who Needs It? *Journal of American Psychoanalytic Association, 29*, 921–938.

Meszaros, I. (2014). *The Necessity of Social Control*. NYU Press.

Möhring, K., Naumann, E., Reifenscheid, M., Wenz, A., Rettig, T., Krieger, U., Friedel, S., Finkel, M., Cornesse, C., Blom, A., & G. (2020). The COVID-19 pandemic and Subjective well-being: Longitudinal Evidence on Satisfaction with Work and Family. *European Societies, 23*, 1–17. https://doi.org/10.1080/14616696.2020.1833066

Monaghan, L. F. (2020). Coronavirus (COVID-19), Pandemic Psychology and Fractured Society: A Sociological Case of Critique Foresight and Action. *Sociology of Health & Illness, 42*(8), 1982–1995.

Monbiot, G. (2020). The Horror Films got It Wrong: This Virus has Turned us into Caring Neighbours. *The Guardian,* March 31. https://www.theguardian.com/commentisfree/2020/mar/31/virus-neighbours-covid-19

Moore, A. (2017). 'Measuring Economic Uncertainty and its Effects'. *Economic Record, 93*(303), 550–575.

Morales- Rodríguez, F. M. (2021). Fear, Stress, Resilience and Coping Strategies during COVID-19 in Spanish University Students. *Sustainability, 13*(11), 2–19.

Nacht, S. (1964). Silence as an Integrative Factor. *International Journal of Psychoanalysis., 45*, 299–303.

Neal, A. G. (1998). *National Trauma and Collective Memory: Major Events in the American Century.* M. E. Sharpe, Armonk.

Nicholson, C. (2010). *Children and Adolescents in Trauma. Creative Therapeutic Approaches* (C. Nicholson, M. Irwin, & K. N. Dwivendi, Eds.). Jessica Kingsley Publishers.

Nicola, M., Alsafi, Z., Sohrabi, C., Kerwan, A., Al-Jabir, A., Iosifidis, C., Agha, M., & Agha, R. (2020). The Socio-economic Implications of the Coronavirus Pandemic (COVID-19): A Review. *International Journal of Surgery, 78*, 185–193.

Nikolo, A. M. (2021). The COVID 19 Pandemic and Individual and Collective Trauma. *International Journal of Applied Psychoanalytic Studies, 1*, 1–6.

Ogden, R. S. (2020). The Passage of Time during the UK Covid-19 Lockdown. *PLoS One, 15*, e0235871. https://doi.org/10.1371/journal.pone.0235871

Okorn, I., Jahović, S., Dobranić-Posavec, M., Mladenović, J., & Glasnović, A. (2020). Isolation in the COVID-19 Pandemic as Re-traumatization of war Experiences. *Croat Med Journal, 61*, 371–376.

Oosterhoff, B., Palmer, C. A., Wilson, J., & Shook, N. (2020). Adolescents' Motivations to Engage in Social Distancing during the COVID-19 Pandemic: Associations with Mental and Social Health. *The Journal of Adolescent Health, 67*, 179–185.

Spini, D., Elcheroth, G., & Fasel, R. (2014). Towards a Community Approach of the Aftermath of War in the Former Yugoslavia: Collective Experiences, Social Practices, and Representations. In D. Spini, G. Elcheroth, & D. C. Biruski (Eds.), *War, Community, and Social Change: Collective Experiences in the Former Yugoslavia.* Springer.

OxCGRT. (2022). Accessed June 15, 2022, from https://ourworldindata.org/covid-stay-home-restrictions#citation

Papadopoulos, R. (2007). Refugees, Trauma and Adversity-Activated Development. *European Journal of Psychotherapy and Counselling, 9*(3), 301–312. https://doi.org/10.1080/13642530701496930

Papadopoulos, R. K. (2004). *Trauma in a Systemic Perspective: Theoretical, Organizational and Clinical Dimensions.* Paper presented at the 14th Congress of the International Family Therapy Association, Istanbul.

Papadopoulos, R. K. (2006). Terrorism and Panic. *Psychotherapy and Politics International, 4*(2), 90–100.

PEP Consolidated Psychoanalytic Glossary. (2016). Produced by: Psychoanalytic Electronic Publishing. https://pep-web.org/browse/document/zbk.069.0000a

Pfefferbaum, B., & North, C. S. (2020). Mental Health and the Covid-19 Pandemic. *The New England Journal of Medicine, 383*(6), 510–512. https://doi.org/10.1056/NEJMp2008017

Pine, F. (1985). *Developmental Theory and Clinical Process.* Yale University Press.

Pinquart, M., & Silbereisen, R. K. (2004). Human Development in Times of Social Change: Theoretical Considerations and Research Needs. *International Journal of Behavioral Development, 28,* 289–298.

Polit, D. F., & Beck, C. T. (2012). *Nursing Research: Generating and Assessing evidence for Nursing Practice* (9th ed.). Lippincott Williams & Wilkins.

Pratt, A. C. (2020). Covid-19 Impacts Cities, cultures and Societies. *City, Culture and Society., 21,* 1–2.

Ren, S. Y., Gao, R. D., & Chen, Y. L. (2020). Fear Can Be More Harmful than the Severe Acute Respiratory Syndrome Coronavirus 2 in Controlling the Coronavirus Disease 2019 Epidemic. *World Journal of Clinical Cases, 8*(4), 652–657.

Ricoeur, P. (1981/2016). *Hermeneutics and the Human Sciences: Essays on Language, Action, and Interpretation.* Cambridge University Press.

Risi, E., Pronzato, R., & Fraia, G. (2020). Everything is Inside the Home: The Boundaries of Home Confinement during the Italian lockdown'. *European Societies, 1–14.* https://doi.org/10.1080/14616696.2020.1828977

Ritchie, J., Lewis, J., McNaughton Nicholls, C., & Ormston, R. (Eds.). (2013). *Qualitative Research Practice. A Guide for Social Science Students and Researchers.* Sage.

Rose, G. J. (1964). Creative Imagination in Terms of Ego 'core' and Boundaries. *International Journal of Psychoanalysis., 45,* 75–84.

Rose, G. J. (1972). Fusion States. In P. L. Giovaccini (Ed.), *Tactics and Techniques in Psychoanalytic Psychotherapy* (pp. 170–188). Science House.

Roseneil, S., & Budgeon, S. (2004). Cultures of Intimacy and Care beyond 'the Family': Personal Life and Social Change in the Early 21st Century. *Current Sociology, 52*(2), 135–159.

Rutter, M. (1994). Stress Research: Accomplishments and Tasks Ahead. In R. J. Haggerty, L. R. Sherrod, N. Garmezy, & M. Rutter (Eds.), *Stress, Risk, and Resilience in Children and Adolescents* (pp. 354–385). Cambridge University Press.

Ryan, G. W., & Bernard, H. R. (2003). Techniques to Identify Themes. *Field Methods, 15*(1), 85–109.

Saul, J. (2013). *Collective Trauma, Collective Healing: Promoting Community Resilience in the Aftermath of Disaster* (Vol. 48). Routledge.

Schaffer, R. (1968). *Aspects of Internalization*. International University Press.

Schejtman, C. R. (2021). Coping with Pandemic, Psychoanalytical Interventions with Parents and Children: Institutional and Community Approaches. *International Journal of Applied Psychoanalytic Studies, 18*(2), 177–187.

Schoon, I. (2007). Adaptations to Changing Times: Agency in Context. *International Journal of Psychology., 42*(2), 94–101.

Sennett, D. (1998). *Der flexible Mensch: Die Kultur des neuen Kapitalismus [The Flexible Person: On the Culture of the New Capitalism]* (8th edn.). Berlin Verlag.

Silbereisen, R. K. (2005). Social Change and Human Development: Experiences from German Unification. *International Journal of Behavioral Development, 29*, 2–13.

Silbereisen, R. K., & Chen, X. (Eds.). (2010). *Social Change and Human Development: Concepts and Results*. Sage.

Silbereisen, R. K., & Eye, A. (1999). *Growing Up in Time of Social Change* (International Studies on Childhood and Adolescence) (Vol. 7). De Gruyter.

Silbereisen, R. K., Pinquart, M., Reitzle, M., Tomasik, M. J., Fabel, K., & Grümer, S. (2006). Psychosocial Resources and Coping with Social Change. http://psydok.psycharchives.de/jspui/bitstream/20.500.11780/460/1/sfb_580_silbereisen_5.pdf

Steiner, J. (1992). The Equilibrium Between the Paranoid-Schizoid and the Depressive Positions. *Clinical Lectures on Klein and Bion, 14*, 46–58.

Stolorow, R. D., & Lachman, F. M. (1980). *Psychoanalysis and Developmental Arrest: Theory and Treatment*. International University Press.

Strong, P. (1990). Epidemic Psychology: A Model. *Sociology of Health and Illness., 12*(3), 249–259.

Tangjia, W. (2014, June). A Philosophical Analysis of the Concept of Crisis. *Frontiers of Philosophy in China, 9*(2), 254–267.

Ungar, M. T. (2004). A Constructionist Discourse on Resilience. *Youth Society, 35*, 341–365.

United Nations Department of Economic and Social Affairs, Islam, S. N., Cheng, H. W. H., Kristinn, Sv, Helgason, K. Sv, Hunt, N., Kawamura, H., LaFleur, M., Iversen, K., & Julca, A. (2021). *UN Department of Economic and Social Affairs (DESA) Working Papers* (18 Jun 2021), 55

Wang, C., Pan, R., Wan, X., Tan, Y., Xu, L., Ho, C. S., & Ho, R. C. (2020). Immediate Psychological Responses and Associated Factors During the Initial Stage of the 2019 Coronavirus Disease (COVID-19) Epidemic among the General Population in China. *International Journal of Environmental Research and Public Health, 17*(5), 1729.

Ward, P. R. (2020). A Sociology of the Covid-19 Pandemic: A Commentary and Research Agenda for Sociologists. *Journal of Sociology*, 1–10. https://doi.org/10.1177/1440783320939682

Watson, M. F., Bacigalupe, G., Daneshpour, M., Han, W. J., & Parra-Cardona, R. (2020). COVID-19 Interconnectedness: Health Inequity, the Climate Crisis, and Collective Trauma. *Family Process, 59*(2), 832–843.

WHO. (2021). World Health Organisation: Social Stigma Associated with COVID-19. Retrieved June 18, 2021, from https://www.who.int/publications/m/item/a-guide-to-preventing-and-addressing-social-stigma-associated-with-covid-19?gclid=CjwKCAjwi_b3BRAGEi-wAemPNUzAjknfOIshPMXXkUYl7xkWVLxvYdtzN8mNiMqswkISRe-MozyhExPhoCw3gQAvD_BwE

Yang, M., He, P., Xu, X., Li, D., Wang, J., Wang, Y., Wang, B., Wang, W., Zhao, M., Lin, H., Deng, M., Deng, T., Kuang, L., & Chen, D. (2021). Disrupted Rhythms of Life, Work and Entertainment and Their Associations with Psychological Impacts under the Stress of the COVID-19 Pandemic: A Survey in 5854 Chinese People with Different Sociodemographic Backgrounds. *PloS one, 16*(5), e0250770. https://doi.org/10.1371/journal.pone.0250770

Zhou, S.-J., Zhang, L.-G., Wang, L.-L., Guo, Z.-C., Wang, J.-Q., Chen, J.-C., Liu, M., Chen, X., & Chen, J.-X. (2020). Prevalence and Socio-demographic Correlates of Psychological Health Problems in Chinese Adolescents During the Outbreak of COVID-19. *European Child & Adolescent Psychiatry, 29*, 749–758.

Žižek, S. (2020). *Pandemic! Covid-19 Shakes the World*. OR Books.